Robotic Donor Nephrectomy

Said Abdallah Al-Mamari
Hervé Quintens
Editors

Robotic Donor Nephrectomy

A Practical Guide

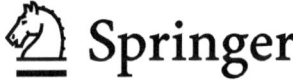 Springer

Editors
Said Abdallah Al-Mamari
Department of Urology
The Royal Hospital
Muscat
Oman

Hervé Quintens
Department of Urology
L'Archet 2 Hospital
University Hospital of Nice
Nice
France

ISBN 978-3-319-04587-0   ISBN 978-3-319-04588-7 (eBook)
DOI 10.1007/978-3-319-04588-7
Springer Cham Heidelberg Dordrecht London New York

Library of Congress Control Number: 2014937324

Printed on acid-free paper

Springer is part of Springer Science+Business Media (www.springer.com)

It is complicated to simplify.
It is simple to complicate.
So there is more merit in the former.

Foreword

Kidney donation by a living relative to a patient with renal failure is an act of extraordinary generosity. The surgeon intervenes in this relationship with care which has developed from the excellent outcomes of this surgical procedure, both in terms of humanity and all aspects of public health.

During this very delicate surgery in which there is no benefit to the donor's health, the surgeon must be at his best technically. Robotic assistance undoubtedly constitutes a significant advance in the minimally invasive laparoscopic approach and adds the possibility of a careful endoscopic procedure with optimal microdissection and hemostasis, **i.e. a minimally invasive technique not only to the abdominal wall (as in standard laparoscopy) but also in the endocorporeal approach.**

The outcome of the surgical procedure is the result of careful preparations. Nowadays preoperative investigations have become more and more accurate both functionally and anatomically. This has allowed precise confirmation of the indications for organ transplantation while being able to anticipate intraoperative difficulties.

The newly standardized technique described in this book by Drs. Al-Mamari and Quintens in a very didactic manner can then be applied to ensure the best chances of success.

Nancy, France   Jacques Hubert

Preface

Kidney transplantation from a living donor provides the best chance for successful renal replacement therapy. However, patient's safety remains of paramount importance and complications are unacceptable. Laparoscopic donor nephrectomy (LDN) has been proven to have a lower surgical mortality and morbidity as well as a lower blood loss, a shorter hospital stay, and a better cosmetic result compared to the open procedure. This has resulted in LDN being considered the standard in many centers. Robot-Assisted Laparoscopic Donor (RALD) nephrectomy is a new trend developed in the last decade. Robotic assistance is increasingly popular worldwide, because it offers optimal operative conditions to the urological surgeon and a shorter learning curve than the standard laparoscopy. The intraoperative technical movements are intuitive with the Endowrist technology of da Vinci Surgical System making suturing easier compared with standard laparoscopy. Robot-assisted surgery allows Urologists to perform more complex procedures with greater precision and confidence, but whether the patient's outcomes are better than in standard laparoscopic approach is still a matter of debate. However there are at least five points which are widely accepted (J. Hubert: Questions d'Actualités; Robotique en 2007. Prog Urol FMC 2007, 2, June 2007, pp 20–23):

1. **Improved ergonomy:** Prevents surgeon's fatigue as well as short and long-term osteo-muscular complaints commonly encountered with the standard laparoscopy

2. **Intuitive movements:** The Endowrist® instruments technology allows the Surgeon to perform quicker and easier movements like dissecting, suturing and knotting
3. **Suppression of tremor:** Ensures safe manipulation of delicate structures in difficult anatomical areas like the renal hilum
4. **Regaining of the hand-eye coordination:** Gives the Surgeon the natural sensation of looking towards his own hands while working, which is lost in standard laparoscopy
5. **Three-dimensional vision:** Provides an unsurpassable view of fine anatomical structures

All these advantages are not insignificant in the setting of a **two-staged delicate surgery** such as donor nephrectomy, in which **the surgeon is dealing with a healthy candidate and harvesting a precious organ for another patient's life.**

In this book, we present well-established multi-ports technique with the da Vinci Surgical System. Novel techniques such as laparo-endoscopic single-site (LESS) surgery and natural orifice transluminal surgery (NOTES) are being developed with the aim at further reducing postoperative pain and length of hospital stay, while offering better cosmetic results.

Muscat, Oman   Said Abdallah Al-Mamari

Acknowledgment

- To **Prof. Jacques Hubert**, HOD Urology Department, University Hospital of Nancy-Brabois, Nancy, France. For his foreword and his accurate remarks and pertinent suggestions which helped to improve the scientific quality of this book.
- To **Dr. Salim Al Busaidy**, HOD Urology Department, the Royal Hospital, Muscat, Oman. For reviewing and amending the text in the English language.
- To **Prof. Jean Amiel**, HOD Urology Department, University Hospital of Nice, Nice, France. For reviewing the content.
- To **Dr. Santhosh Narayana**, Urology Department, The Royal Hospital, Muscat, Oman. For his active participation in the bibliographic references.
- To **Melissa Morton, Julia Megginson, and Suganya Selvaraj**, for their fruitful collaboration in the final presentation of this book.

Contents

1 Surgical Anatomy of the Retroperitoneum . . . .　1
Said Abdallah Al-Mamari and Jacques Jourdan

2 Pre-operative Investigations . . . .　11
Said Abdallah Al-Mamari and Jacques Jourdan

**3 Anesthesiological Aspects Relevant for
Robotic Assisted Laparoscopic Donor
Nephrectomy** . . . .　17
Said Abdallah Al-Mamari and Bruno Malzac

4 Robotic Instruments . . . .　27
Said Abdallah Al-Mamari and Hervé Quintens

5 Surgical Steps . . . .　35
Said Abdallah Al-Mamari and Hervé Quintens

Index . . . .　85

Contributors

Said Abdallah Al-Mamari Department of Urology, The Royal Hospital, Muscat, Oman

Jacques Jourdan Department of Urology, L'Archet 2 Hospital, University Hospital of Nice, Nice, France

Bruno Malzac Department of Anesthesiology, L'Archet 2 Hospital, University Hospital of Nice, Nice, France

Hervé Quintens Department of Urology, L'Archet 2 Hospital, University Hospital of Nice, Nice, France

Chapter 1
Surgical Anatomy of the Retroperitoneum

Said Abdallah Al-Mamari and Jacques Jourdan

The boundaries of the **retroperitoneum** are:

- Posteriorly: The posterior abdominal wall, made of the lumbar vertebral column medially, and the **psoas** and quadratus lumborum muscles laterally.
- Anteriorly: The posterior parietal peritoneum along with intra-peritoneal organs which are fixed to it.
- Cranially: The diaphragm muscle.
- Caudally: The extraperitoneal pelvic structures (urinary bladder etc.).

The contents are:

- Medially: The **abdominal aorta**, the **inferior Vena Cava**, the peri-aortic autonomic nerve plexuses, the lumbo-aortic lymphatic vessels, the **duodenum**, and the head of the pancreas.

S.A. Al-Mamari (✉)
Department of Urology, The Royal Hospital,
Muscat, Oman
e-mail: sabdal67@yahoo.com

J. Jourdan
Department of Urology, L'Archet 2 Hospital,
University Hospital of Nice, Nice, France

S.A. Al-Mamari, H. Quintens (eds.), *Robotic Donor Nephrectomy*, DOI 10.1007/978-3-319-04588-7_1,
© Springer International Publishing Switzerland 2014

1

- Laterally: **The kidneys and their vessels, the adrenals, the ureters, the gonadal vessels,** the body and tail of pancreas, and the **ascending and descending colons**.

  – **The psoas major muscle** originates from the 12th thoracic and the five lumbar vertebrae. In about half of the population a smaller psoas minor can be seen medially to the psoas major [1]. Both psoas muscles are covered by the psoas fascia. Caudally they fuse with the iliacus muscle to insert into the lesser trochanter of femur. The psoas muscles are surgically important because the kidneys and the upper 2/3 of the ureters lie on them.
  – **The kidneys** are in contact with the diaphragm muscle posteriorly which covers their upper third with the 12th rib crossing at the lower extent of this muscle. The lower two thirds of each kidney lie medially on the psoas muscle, while the quadratus lumborum and the aponeurosis of the transversus abdominis muscle are seen more laterally. Anteriorly, the **right kidney** is in contact with the liver cranially, to whom it is attached by the **hepatorenal ligament**, and with the right adrenal gland, medially with the **descending duodenum** which is also in close relation with the hilar structures, and anteriorly with the **hepatic flexure of the colon** in contact with the kidney lower pole. To fully visualize the upper pole of the right kidney, it is usually necessary for the surgeon to divide the right triangular and part of the anterior coronary ligaments which fix the liver to the inferior surface of the diaphragm. **The left kidney** is in relation superiorly with the tail of the pancreas and the splenic vessels, the left adrenal gland, and the spleen to whom it is attached by the **splenorenal ligament**. The importance of this ligament lies on that the splenic capsule can be accidentally torn by an excessive downward pressure on the left kidney. Caudally, the kidney is in contact with the **splenic flexure of the colon**. The phreno-colic, the spleno-colic, and the spleno-renal ligaments are found in this area and have to be divided to allow visualization of the left kidney upper pole.

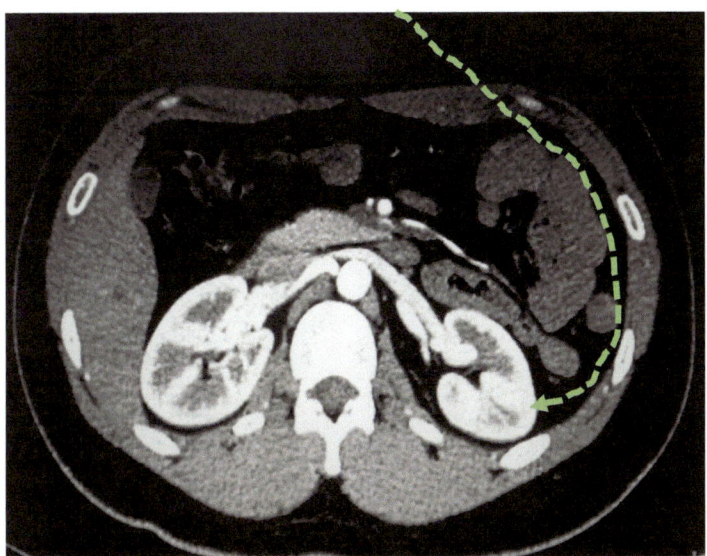

FIGURE 1.1 Contrast-CT of the abdomen. The *dotted line* shows the schematic pathway of intraperitoneal laparoscopic left nephrectomy. However, this *curved line* is in reality straightened by the lateral position of the patient lying on the opposite side and the fall of the colon medially after Toldt's fascia is incised

Because of the above mentioned anatomical relations to both kidneys, it is of **paramount importance to mobilize the colon and its mesentery** for exposing the kidneys and ureters via an intraperitoneal approach (Fig. 1.1).

- **The renal arteries** arise laterally from the aorta at L2 level, immediately below the origin of the **superior mesenteric artery**. Renal artery originating from the level of L1–L2 intervertebral disc has been observed in 37.0 % and 38.9 % of cases on the right and left sides, respectively [2]. The right renal artery courses **behind the inferior vena cava** to join the corresponding kidney while the left renal artery joins directly the left kidney. At the renal hilum, they lie between the **renal veins**

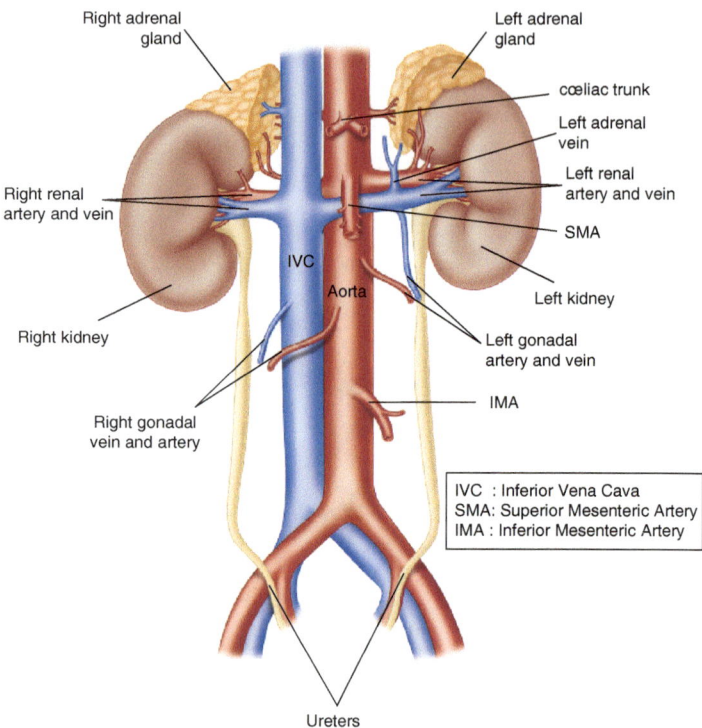

FIGURE 1.2 Retroperitoneum: kidneys, ureters, adrenals and great vessels

anteriorly and the **renal pelves** posteriorly; the mnemonic **VAP** (Vein-Artery-Pelvis) refers to this topography from anterior to posterior. **The left renal vein crosses the aorta anteriorly** to join the vena cava. During its course, it passes between the aorta and **the first few centimeters of the superior mesenteric artery** (SMA) originating from the anterior aspect of the aorta (Fig. 1.2). This position exposes the left renal vein to the rare **entrapment or nutcracker syndrome** between the aorta and the SMA. **The left renal vein is typically longer than the right** measuring 6–10 and 2–4 cm respectively. This is the reason why the left kidney is

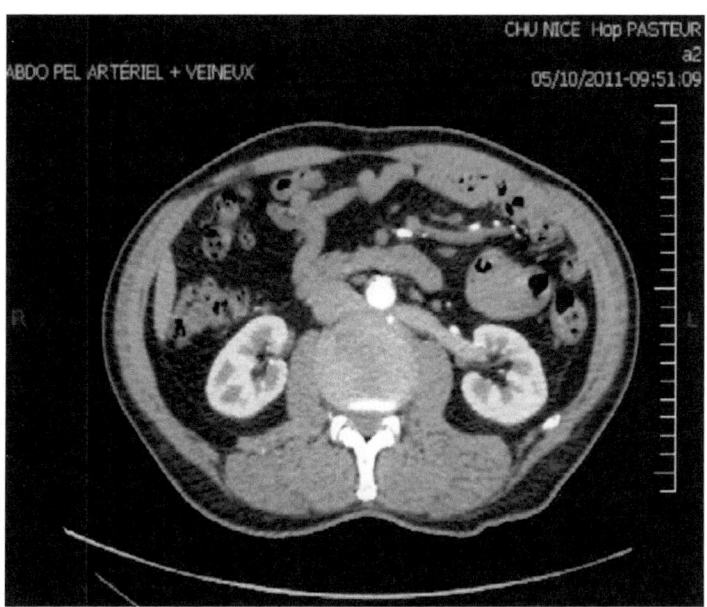

Figure 1.3 Retroaortic left renal vein

more frequently preferred for a transplantation procedure. **The left renal vein receives the left adrenal vein superiorly, one or two lumbar veins posteriorly, and the left gonadal vein inferiorly, while its right counterpart does not receive any tributaries. Anatomical variations** of the renal vasculature are common, occurring in 25–40 % of kidneys, and may exist in **multiple renal arteries** (up to 5!) mostly on the left side [1], and **retroaortic** (Fig. 1.3) **or circumaortic left renal vein**. It is not uncommon to see a lumbar vein joining the gonadal vein just before it enters the renal vein. Supernumerary veins are less commonly encountered, and occur mostly on the right side. It is also common to see early division of the renal arteries. More rarely found is a precaval right renal artery and a **duplicated Inferior Vena Cava** [3] (Fig. 1.4). When lower pole arteries are present, it is

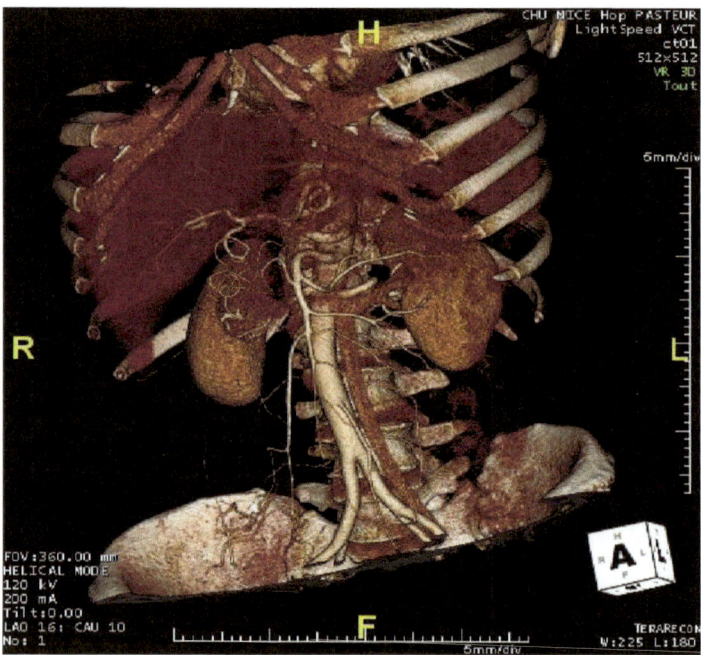

FIGURE 1.4 Duplicated inferior vena cava: the left root runs along the left aortic border and crosses at the renal hilum level to join the right counterpart

of surgical importance to remember their **tendency to cross anterior to the IVC on the right side and anterior to the collecting system on either side**, eventually causing a pelvi-ureteric junction obstruction.

- The **adrenal glands** measure 3–5 cm for an approximate weight of 5 g. They are bright orange in color and are easily differentiated from the pale yellow fatty renal fascia. Each gland is situated in the upper pole of the corresponding kidney with which it is enclosed in a common **perirenal (Gerota's) fascia**, with only a layer of connective tissue separating the two organs. The right adrenal gland is pyramidal in shape and is more superiorly located than the crescentric left one (Fig. 1.2). The left adrenal vein drains into the superior aspect of the renal vein, while the right one drains directly into the IVC.

– The **ureters** descend from the renal pelves posterior to the renal arteries and veins and lie posteriorly on the psoas muscles. Anteriorly, the right ureter is in contact with the ascending colon, the caecum and the colonic mesentery, the left one is related to the descending colon, the sigmoid and their mesenteries. **On both sides, at the junction between its first and second third, the ureter is crossed anteriorly by the gonadal vessels which pass from medial cranially to lateral caudally** (Fig. 1.2). Inferiorly, the ureters enter the true pelvis by passing in front of the iliac vessels, generally at the division of the common iliac into internal and external iliac vessels. **In females, the distal ureters are crossed anteriorly by the uterine arteries in close relationship with the uterine cervix**. This make them particularly exposed to injury during hysterectomy.

– The **gonadal (testicular or ovarian) arteries** arise from the aorta below the origin of the renal arteries. In both sexes, the **right gonadal artery crosses anterior to the inferior vena cava. In men, it then crosses over the ureter and enter the internal inguinal ring to exit the retroperitoneum, while in women it crosses medially back over the external iliac vessels and enters the pelvis.** Caudally, the **gonadal veins** have a course similar to gonadal arteries. But cranially **they stay more laterally and lie closer to the ipsilateral ureter**. The terminal drainage varies with the side: the right **gonadal vein draining directly into the anterior aspect of the IVC below the level of the renal vein, while the left terminates into the inferior aspect of the ipsilateral renal vein** (Fig. 1.2). The terminations of the left gonadal and adrenal veins at the left renal vein form a **violet cross,** a key-point to identify in every transperitoneal laparoscopic left nephrectomy. The importance of recognizing the termination of the right gonadal vein on the IVC avoids the risk of injury while dissecting the IVC anteriorly in an attempt to locate the right renal vein. In a small minority of patients the right gonadal vein can enter the right renal vein rather than the IVC [3]. Another rare anatomical variation occurs when a lumbar vein joins the posterior aspect of the right renal vein instead of joining the IVC directly.

- **The perirenal or Gerota's fascia** envelops the kidneys (with the perirenal fat) and the adrenals on all aspects except inferiorly, where it remains open leaving a potential space in which urine or pus can spread along the psoas muscle when perirenal extravasation or abscesses form [1]. Certain anatomists refer to the thinner anterior lamina of the Gerota's fascia as the Toldt's membrane and the thicker posterior one as the Zuckerkandl's fascia [4].

- The paracolic fascia, also called **Toldt's fascia,** fixes both ascending and descending colons to the postero-lateral abdominal wall**.** At its lateral reflection on the abdominal wall, the fascia forms the avascular **white line of Toldt** which is incised in order to release the colon from the abdominal wall to enter the retroperitoneum.

References

1. Kyle Anderson J, Kabalin JN, Cadeddu JA. Surgical anatomy of the retroperitoneum, adrenals, kidneys, and ureters. In: Wein AJ, Kavoussi LR, Novick AC, Partin AW, Peters CA, editors. Campbell-Walsh urology. 9th ed. Philadelphia: Saunders Elsevier; 2007. p. 3–5, 20–30, and 34–7.
2. Gümüş H, Bükte Y, Ozdemir E, Cetinçakmak MG, Tekbaş G, Ekici F, Onder H, Uyar A. Variations of renal artery in 820 patients using 64-detector CT-angiography. Ren Fail. 2012;34: 286–90.
3. Apisarnthanarak P, Suvannarerg V, Muangsomboon K, Taweemonkongsap T, Hargrove NS. Renal vascular variants in living related renal donors: evaluation with CT angiography. J Med Assoc Thai. 2012;95:941–8.

4. Blute ML, Brant Inman SR. Anatomy and principles of renal surgery: In: Smith JA Jr., Howards SS, McGuire EJ. Preminger GM. Hinman's atlas of urologic surgery. 3rd ed. Saunders, Elsevier: 2012. p. 967–970.

Further Reading

Carola R, Harley JP, Noback CR. Human anatomy and physiology. New York: McGraw-Hill, Inc.; 1990. p. 767–9.

McMinn RMH. Last's anatomy. 9th ed. Edinburgh: Churchill Livingstone; 1995. p. 366–8 and 371–2.

Snell RS. Clinical anatomy for medical students. 5th ed. Philadelphia: Lippincott Williams & Wilkins; 1995. p. 224–30.

Tortora GJ, Grabowski SR. Principles of anatomy and physiology. 8th ed. San Francisco: Harper Collins College Publishers; 1996. p. 848–52.

Williams PL, Bannister LH, Berry MM, et al. Gray's Anatomy, 38th ed. Edinburgh: Churchill Livingstone, 1995. p. 1815–9.

Chapter 2
Pre-operative Investigations

Said Abdallah Al-Mamari and Jacques Jourdan

A suitable candidate for kidney donation is usually seen 1–3 months before the date of surgery. He is assessed by Nephrologists, Urological Surgeons and Anesthetists, by thorough investigations with the aim of avoiding surgery for any person who is ASA 3 or above. Moreover, although we haven't faced obese candidates in our experience, we think that a BMI above 35 should be considered a relative contra-indication for kidney donation since those subjects would be more exposed to perioperative complications and late renal dysfunction.

Approval by a Cardiologist is mandatory for donors aged above 40 years, and should be supported by full investigations including echocardiography, stress coronary reserve measurements, and if necessary coronary angiography, **since morbidity and mortality are not acceptable for a living donor.**

Radiological examinations include a **multidetector-row computerized tomography (MDCT)-renal angiography** (Fig. 2.1) and a **technetium-99 m mercaptoacetyltriglycine renography**

S.A. Al-Mamari (✉)
Department of Urology, The Royal Hospital,
Muscat, Oman
e-mail: sabdal67@yahoo.com

J. Jourdan
Department of Urology, L'Archet 2 Hospital,
University Hospital of Nice, Nice, France

S.A. Al-Mamari, H. Quintens (eds.), *Robotic Donor Nephrectomy*, DOI 10.1007/978-3-319-04588-7_2,
© Springer International Publishing Switzerland 2014

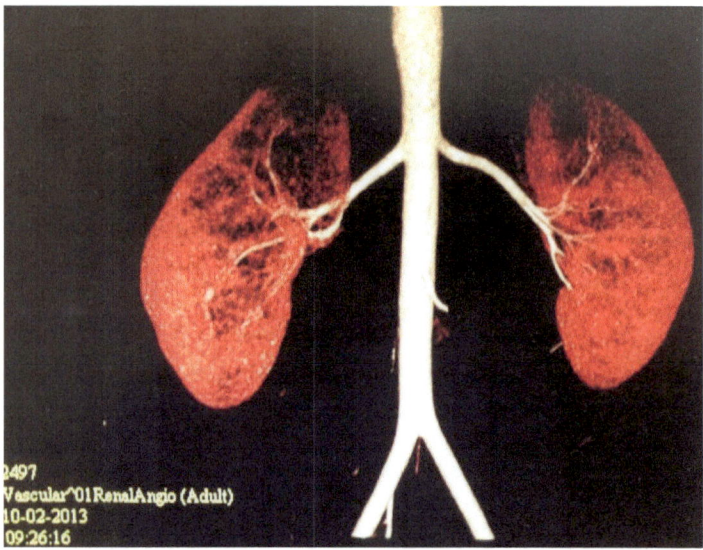

FIGURE 2.1 Renal CT-angiography showing the commonest finding of bilateral single renal artery

(^{99m}Tc-MAG3) to assess the renal split function and provide at the same time informations about the excretory phase.

The primary role of the CT-angiography is to depict the vasculature of the kidneys since renal vascular anatomical variants are common [1]. The presence of 2–3 renal arteries does not preclude kidney donation but constitute an additional stress to both the kidney harvesting and the transplantation techniques (Fig. 2.2a, b). For the interest of this subject, we have chosen such a case in our description of the left nephrectomy. Many techniques have been described to avoid the need for a time consuming and stressful double arterial

FIGURE 2.2 (**a**) CT-Angiography scan of the donor kidneys showing two arteries on the left side. Note the crossing-over resulting in the cranial artery supplying the lower half of the kidney and the caudal artery supplying the upper half. (**b**) Bilateral multiple renal arteries

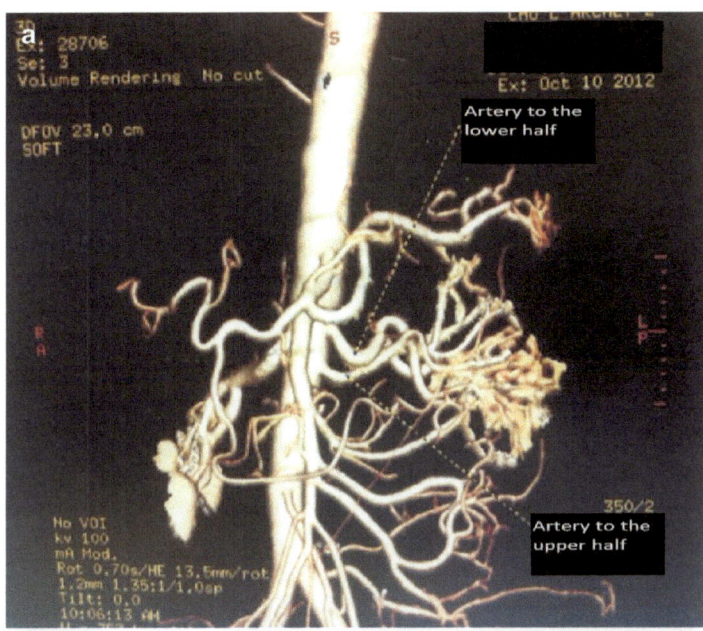

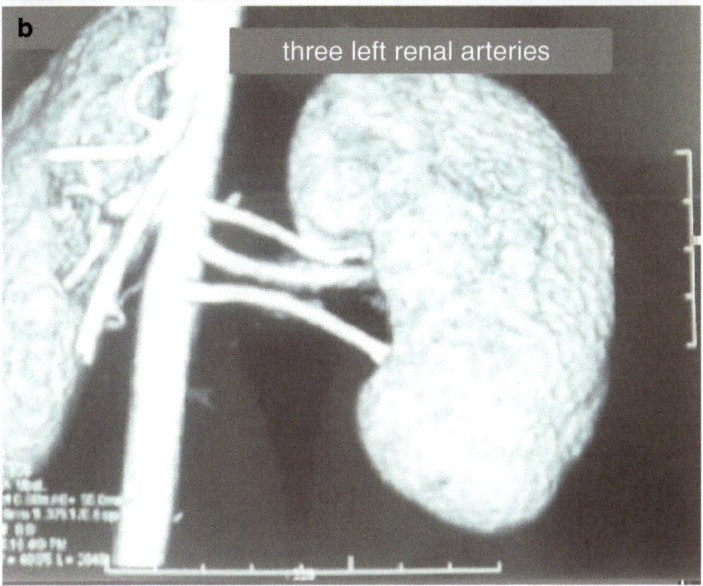

anastomosis in the recipient, including a Y-technique and a double gun-barrel fashion, however their description is beyond the scope of this book. On the other hand, it is generally accepted that the presence of more than three renal arteries is a contraindication for donor nephrectomy, and every effort should be made to find a "better" donor if the contralateral kidney does not offer a feasible vascular anatomy. CT-angiography allows one to exclude vascular abnormalities which constitute a contraindication to the living donor nephrectomy: renal artery stenosis and aneurysm, and fibromuscular dysplasia. The venous anatomy is equally important to be known and CT-angiography may reveal unusual presentation such as a retroaortic or a circumaortic left renal vein, both of which being manageable without much difficulty once anticipated. Axial CT-angiograms analysis allows also one to define the reno-azygo-lumbar venous arch and to be more cautious during dissection of the left renal vein inferior and posterior aspects.

Other benefits of the CT-angiography include visualizing the anatomy of the collecting systems and ureters, and detecting renal parenchymal abnormalities such as atrophy, cysts, scars, and tumors. It may also reveal renal stones, and extrarenal pathology, e.g. adrenal or gastro-intestinal tumors, inflammatory bowel disease, etc [2]. The tomodensitometry scan provides also an accurate evaluation of the kidneys volume which may show discrepancy with the values obtained from isotope renograms. Being projectional, the latter studies may indeed underestimate the function of a malrotated kidney, especially the right one.

There is no universal cut off value for split function in the evaluation of living kidney donors. However it is usual in many institutions to exclude candidates with unequal relative functions beyond 60/40 % [3]. When the split functions are within the ranges 40–47/53–60 %, the less functioning unit is harvested to avoid renal function impairment in the healthy donor. When the relative function of the kidneys is equal, i.e. within 48 and 52 % range, the left kidney is preferred for donation because of its longer vein, unless arterial anatomy favors the right one.

References

1. Apisarnthanarak P, Suvannarerg V, Muangsomboon K, Taweemonkongsap T, Hargrove NS. Renal vascular variants in living related renal donors: evaluation with CT angiography. J Med Assoc Thai. 2012;95:941–8.
2. Chu LC, Sheth S, Segev DL, Montgomery RA, Fishman EK. Role of MDCT angiography in selection and presurgical planning of potential renal donors. AJR Am J Roentgenol. 2012;199:1035–41.
3. Adam L. Summerlin, Mark E. Lockhart, Andrew M. Strang, Peter N. Kolettis, Naomi S. Fineberg, and J. Kevin Smith. Determination of Split Renal Function by 3D Reconstruction of CT Angiograms: A Comparison to Gamma Camera Renography. AJR Am J Roentgenol. 2008;191:1552–8.

Further Reading

Abutaleb N. Is the omission of assessing split renal function from living kidney donor's work-up justified? Letter to the Editor. Saudi J Kidney Dis Transpl. 2010;21:350–3.

Grewal GS, Blake GM. Reference data for 51Cr-EDTA measurements of the glomerular filtration rate derived from live kidney donors. Nucl Med Commun. 2005;26:61–5.

Renard-Penna R, Ayed A, Barrou B, Grenier P. Pre-kidney-transplant evaluation of donors and recipients. J Radiol. 2011;92:358–66.

Summerlin AL, Lockhart ME, Strang AM, Kolettis PN, Fineberg NS, Kevin Smith J. Determination of split renal function by 3D reconstruction of CT angiograms: a comparison to gamma camera renography. AJR Am J Roentgenol. 2008;191:1552–8.

Tombul ST, Aki FT, Gunay M, Inci K, Hazirolan T, Karcaaltincaba M, Erkan I, Bakkaloglu A, Yasavul U, Bakkaloglu M. Preoperative evaluation of hilar vessel anatomy with 3-D computerized tomography in living kidney donors. Transplant Proc. 2008;40:47–9.

.

Chapter 3
Anesthesiological Aspects Relevant for Robotic Assisted Laparoscopic Donor Nephrectomy

Said Abdallah Al-Mamari and Bruno Malzac

The patient is admitted the day before surgery and blood investigations are repeated for Hb, renal function tests, and coagulation profile. **HLA cross-match tests are also repeated** to rule out antibodies which may have been newly formed by the recipient during recent hemodialysis sessions, through blood transfusion, or spontaneously. Blood grouping is performed, irregular agglutinins are ruled out, and two blood units are arranged and kept in the hospital blood bank only to be brought in the operating theatre (OT) if needed. During the evening ward round, the candidate is again seen by the Nephrologists, Surgeons, and Anesthetists; he is informed about the forthcoming procedures, and an inform consent is taken. Thromboprophylaxy is started with a subcutaneous low molecular weight heparin and continued for about 4 weeks. Here the most commonly used drug is Enoxaparin (Clexane®, Lovenox®) 40 mg once a day. Alternatively Nadroparin (Fraxiparine®), or Dalteparin

S.A. Al-Mamari (✉)
Department of Urology, The Royal Hospital, Muscat, Oman
e-mail: sabdal67@yahoo.com

B. Malzac
Department of Anesthesiology, L'Archet 2 Hospital,
University Hospital of Nice, Nice, France

S.A. Al-Mamari, H. Quintens (eds.), *Robotic Donor Nephrectomy*, DOI 10.1007/978-3-319-04588-7_3,
© Springer International Publishing Switzerland 2014

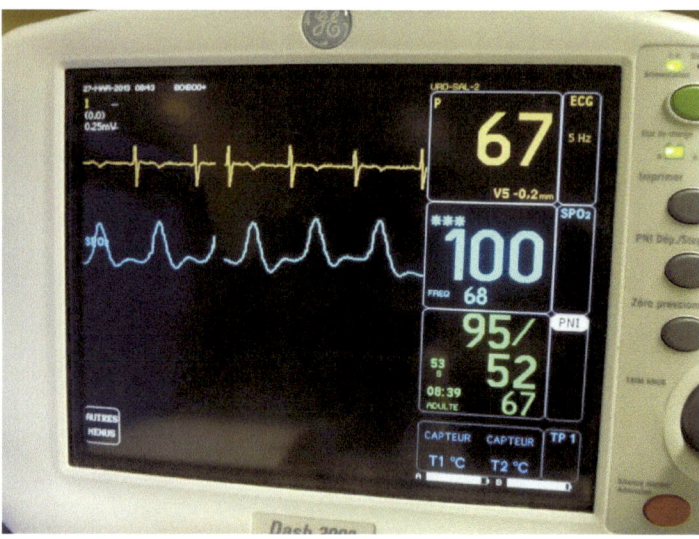

FIGURE 3.1 Non-invasive monitoring of vital parameters

(Fragmin®) can also be used. A bath is taken before sleeping and the patient remains nil by mouth after midnight.

After taking another bath in the early morning, the patient is shaved from the midline to the corresponding flank and inferiorly beyond the level of the Pfannenstiel site. He wears anti-embolism compression stockings, commonly referred to as ThromboEmbolism-Deterrent (TED) hose, and receives a premedication based on 5 mg sub/lingual Midazolam (Hypnovel®, Dormicum®) or 50 mg oral Hydroxyzine (Atarax®, Vistaril®) 30–60 min before being transferred into the OT department. The donor is always the first on the OT list and the operating room is cleaned and prepared from the evening before the surgery.

In the OT, non-invasive monitoring is initiated to observe routine parameters like the blood pressure, the heart rate, the O_2 saturation and the ECG (Fig. 3.1). The patient is covered with forced-air warming blankets and perfused with a slow 0.9 % NaCl solution to maintain a peripheral venous access.

The induction is done only in the presence of the Surgeon. In Nice University Hospital it is performed according to the

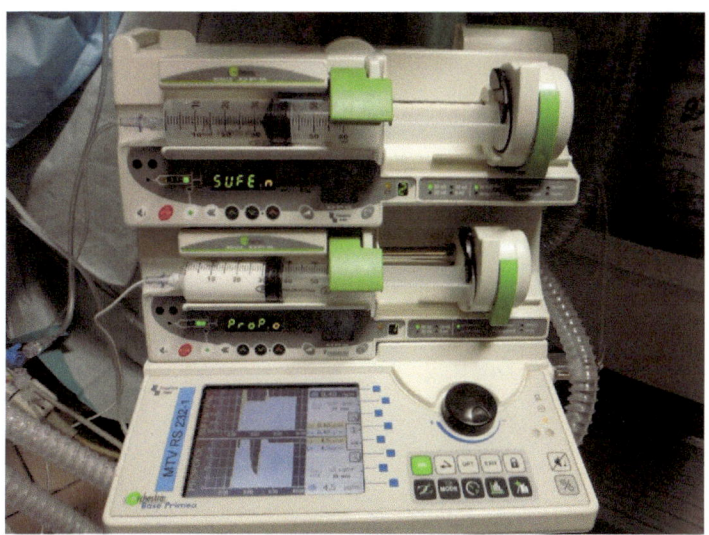

FIGURE 3.2 Target-Controlled Intravenous anesthesia (TCI) technique

Target-Controlled *Intravenous anesthesia (TCI)* technique (or AIVOC in French: Anesthésie Intra-Veineuse à Objectif de Concentration). The technique involves the use of an electrical syringe with a computer-controlled administration rate, according to an accurate calculation based on patient's weight, age, height, and sex. Drugs commonly used by TCI technique are: Propofol (Diprivan®) 2.5 to 6 µg/ml (cerebral target) and Sufentanil (Sufenta®) 0.2 to 0.5 ng/ml (cerebral target) (Fig. 3.2). A prophylactic antibiotic is given on induction and consists of a second generation cephalosporin: Cefazolin 2 g or Cefuroxime 1.5 g single dose.

Curarisation is achieved by giving a 0.5 mg/Kg Atracurium besylate bolus. When enough curarisation depth is reached as shown in a special monitor, maintenance is obtained with 0.3–0.5 mg/Kg/h (Fig. 3.3).

Ventilation is delivered with the aid of a mask aiming an Oxygen FiO_2 of 100 % (Fig. 3.4).

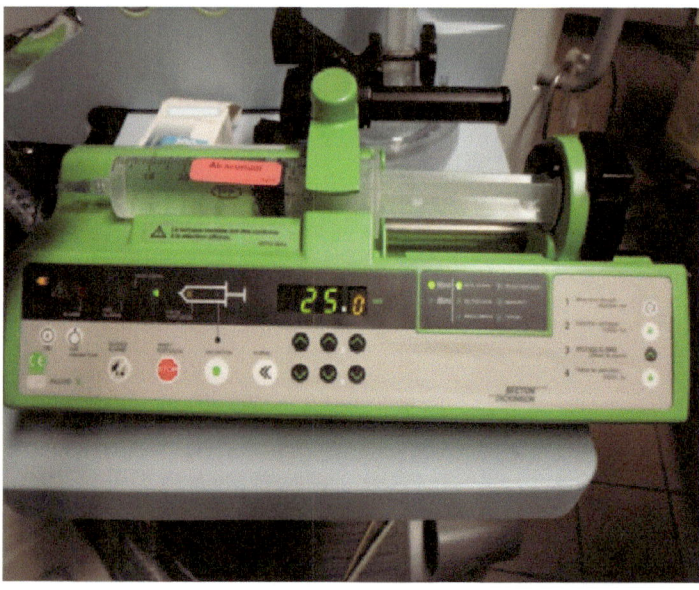

FIGURE 3.3 Curarisation pump

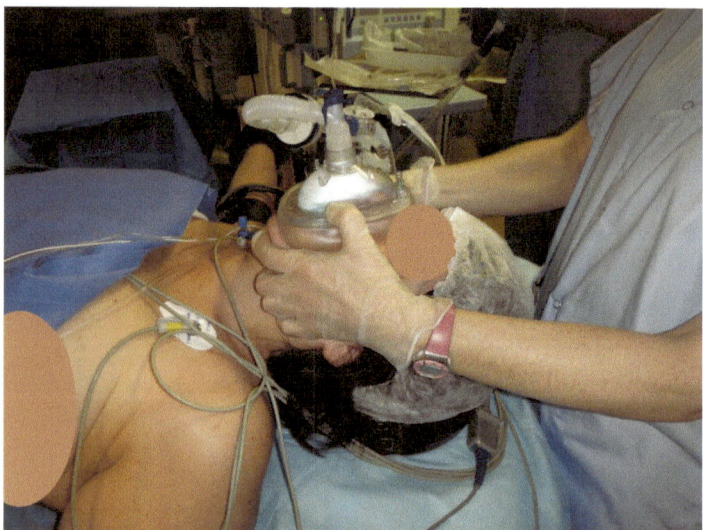

FIGURE 3.4 Patient ventilated with the aid of a mask

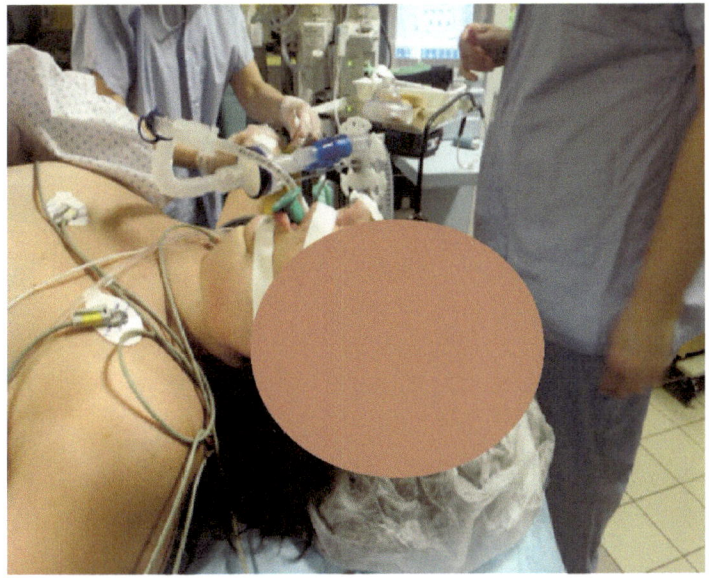

FIGURE 3.5 Patient intubated and ventilated

Once curarisation and TCI targets are achieved, the patient is intubated and ventilated (Fig. 3.5).

A vitamin A solution is instillated on the corneas and the eye-lids are occluded with a tape.

At this time a second peripheral line is inserted for security purpose, in order to anticipate any intraoperative surgical complication (bleeding etc.), the first perfusion line being reserved for the TCI drugs administration. A **central venous line is not needed since the patient is not at high risk**. An indwelling (generally no 16 French) Foley's catheter is inserted to keep the urinary bladder empty, as well as an oro-gastric Ryle's tube to decompress the stomach.

Positioning of the patient on the operating table is adjusted and finalized in accordance with the surgeon. The patient is put in a **semi-lateral position with side of the kidney to be harvested up, and the back turned to the robotic cart.** The insulating diathermy pad is attached to the lateral aspect of the upper thigh (Fig. 3.6). The lower leg is flexed and a pillow

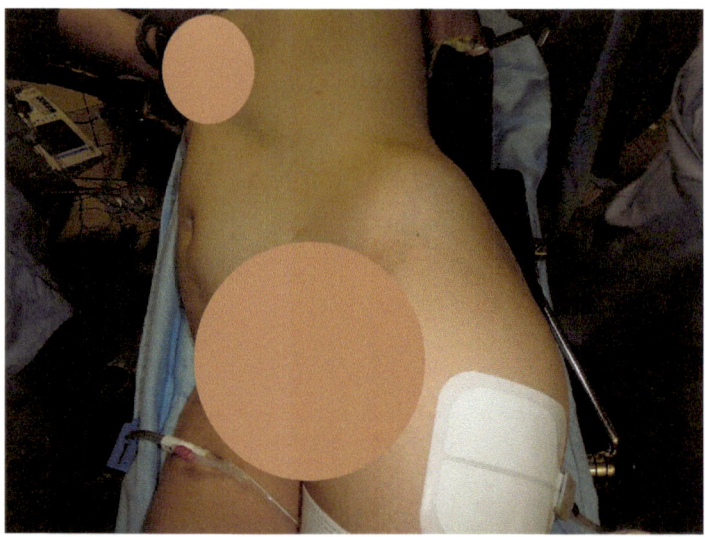

FIGURE 3.6 Patient in a semi-lateral position

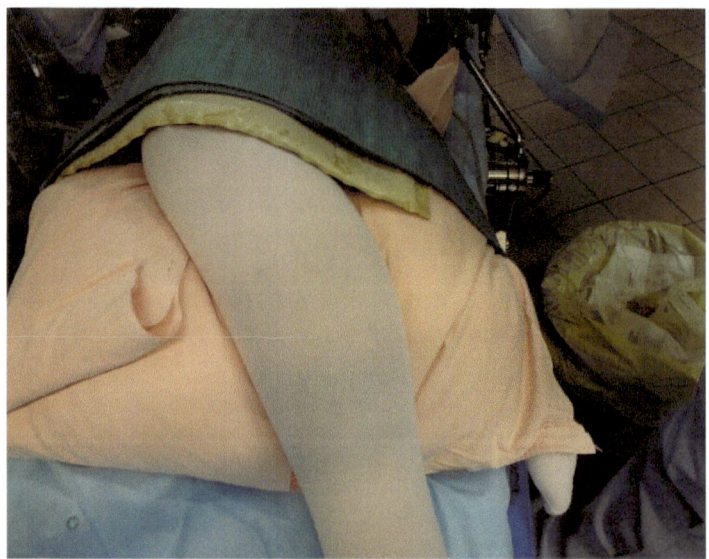

FIGURE 3.7 Cushion between the flexed lower and the upper legs

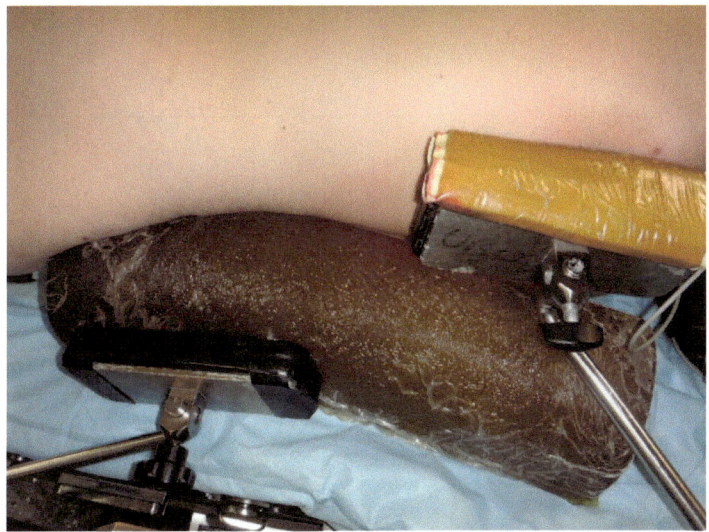

FIGURE 3.8 Padded supports on the patient's back

is positioned between the two legs. Cushions and pads are used to protect all pressure areas including the knees, elbows, ankles and hips (Figs. 3.7 and 3.8).

Once correctly positioned, the patient's chest and head are covered with warming-sheets (Figs. 3.9 and 3.10) and surgery can begin.

The transient laparoscopy-related effects of the pneumo-peritoneum are carefully observed:

- Decreased lung compliance and reduced tidal volume
- Compressed basal alveoli by the elevated diaphragm
- Decrease venous return which reduces the cardiac output, then the blood pressure.
- Oliguria (generally unnoticed).

A special monitor reveals the ventilatory parameters at real time (Fig. 3.11).

To address the hypercapnia, alveolar ventilation is improved in two ways:

- by increasing the Inspiratory time in the I:E cycle bringing it from a normal 1:2 to a nearly 1:1 ratio.

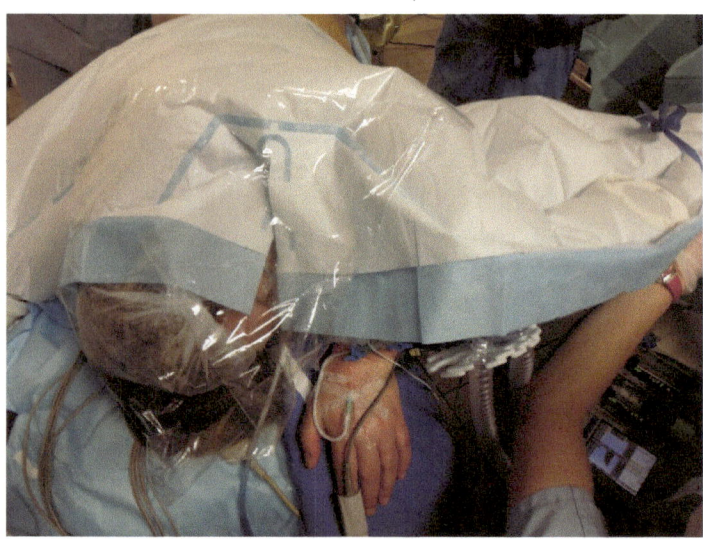

FIGURE 3.9 Patient's chest and head covered with warming sheets

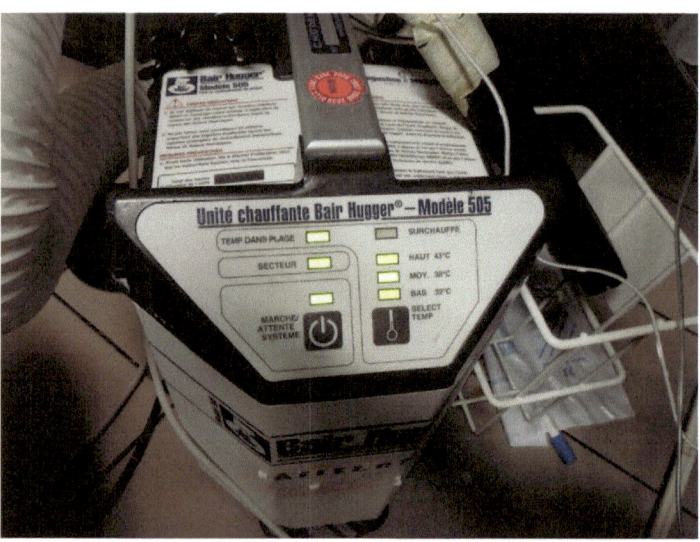

FIGURE 3.10 Warming unit

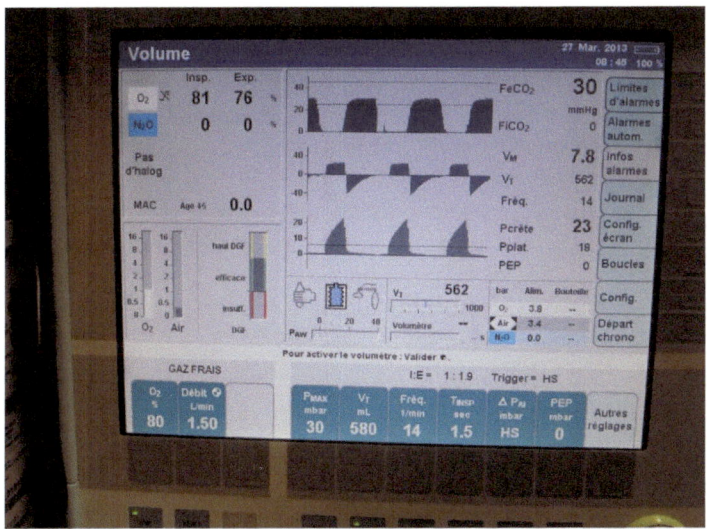

FIGURE 3.11 Monitoring of the ventilatory parameters

- by increasing the respiratory frequency since one cannot increase the tidal volume in the presence of pneumoperitoneum.

The kidney donor is specifically perfused with 9 % NaCl, or with natural colloids (e.g. 4 % Albumin); starch-based artificial colloids should be avoided due to their tendency to accumulate in the renal interstitium, inducing a tubulopathy and potential renal failure.

After surgery, the patient is kept intubated and shifted to the recovery room, where he is laid in a bed, monitored, and warmed.

When ear thermometer indicates a body temperature above 36 °C, and no surgical complication is present, extubation is performed usually after about 30–60 min of monitoring in the recovery room. The Ryle's tube is removed at the same time.

Post-operative analgesia is administered using a 6-hourly i-v 1 g Paracetamol (Perfalgan®) and a 24- h preloaded i-v electrical syringe containing 240 mg Phloroglucinol (spas-fon®), 300 mg Tramadol (Contramal®), 100 mg Nefopam (Acupan®). 2.5 mg Droperidol (Droleptan®) is also included in this cocktail to prevent nausea. A morphine-based patient-controlled analgesia (PCA) is associated to this protocol in case of severe pain.

The patient is taken back to the ward in the high dependency area for 24 h. He is then transferred to normal rooms/beds from day 2 if no complication arises. The urinary catheter is removed the morning of day 2 and the patient is encouraged to walk.

From day 2, Paracetamol is continued and other drugs are administered only when indicated. Oral intake is allowed after flatus emission, and the patient is discharged home from day 3 to day 5 post-operatively. Generally the patient will be able to resume normal professional activities after a sick leave of 2 weeks.

Further Reading

Billard V, Cazalaà JB, Servin F, Viviand X. Target-controlled intravenous anesthesia. Ann Fr Anesth Reanim. 1997;16:250–73.

Jaoua H, Zghidi S, Askri A, Jendoubi A, Ammar N, Lassili S, Laaribi W, Darmoul S, Khelifi S, Ben FK. Target-controlled intravenous anesthesia during laparoscopic surgery for obesity. Tunis Med. 2011;89:37–42.

Chapter 4
Robotic Instruments

Said Abdallah Al-Mamari and Hervé Quintens

Below is a non-exhaustive list of the most commonly used robotic instruments in abdominal surgery. In our experience, we use only the items in **bold** for donor nephrectomy. For the sake of completeness, we also present the equivalent items which are used for pelvic surgeries (cystectomy and prostatectomy).

1. 8-mm instruments (to be used through 10 mm ports)

   - EndoWrist® needle-holders: **Large Needle Driver** (Fig. 4.1).
   - EndoWrist® Graspers: **Prograsp™** (Fig. 4.2), Cadiere Forceps (Fig. 4.3), or Double Fenestrated Graspers.
   - EndoWrist® Monopolar Cautery Instruments: **Hot Shears™ (Monopolar Curved Scissors)** (Fig. 4.4), and **Permanent Cautery Hook** (Fig. 4.5).

S.A. Al-Mamari (✉)
Department of Urology, The Royal Hospital,
Muscat, Oman
e-mail: sabdal67@yahoo.com

H. Quintens
Department of Urology, L'Archet 2 Hospital,
University Hospital of Nice, Nice, France

S.A. Al-Mamari, H. Quintens (eds.), *Robotic Donor Nephrectomy*, DOI 10.1007/978-3-319-04588-7_4,
© Springer International Publishing Switzerland 2014

- EndoWrist® Bipolar Cautery Instruments: **PreCise™ Bipolar Forceps** (Fig. 4.6), Maryland Bipolar Forceps (Fig. 4.7), PK® Dissecting Bipolar Forceps, or Fenestrated Bipolar Forceps.
- Ultrasonic Energy Instruments (optional): Harmonic® Curved Shears.
- EndoWrist® Clip Appliers (optional): Small Clip Applier and Large Hem-O-lok® Clip Applier.
- Accessories: **Cannulas, Obturators and Seals** (Fig. 4.8).

2. **3-D vision camera and Endoscope**, **0°** and 30° (Figs. 4.9 and 4.10) (through a 12 mm port)
3. Manually controlled instruments (by the assistant)**: Suction device, Hem-o-Lok® clip appliers** (through a 12 mm port) (Fig. 4.11)**, 15-mm Endocatch™** (through the Pfannenstiel incision)
4. Full laparoscopic conversion table is always kept ready and covered with a sterile drape (Fig. 4.12).

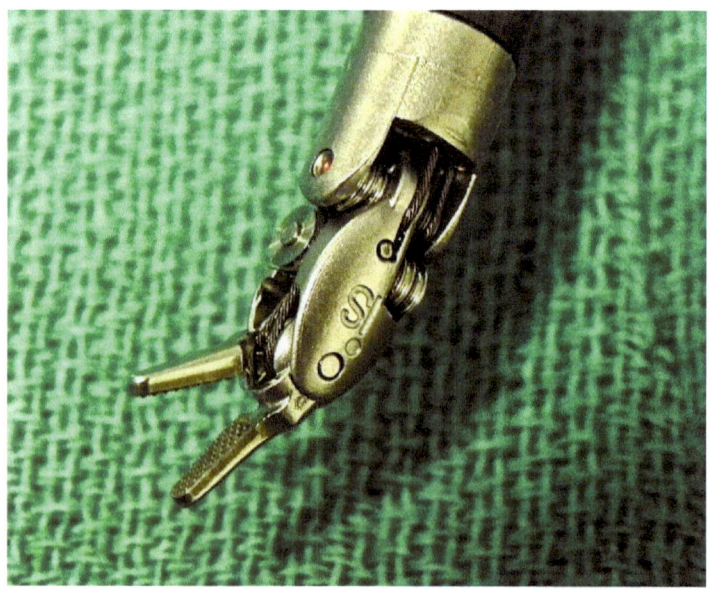

FIGURE 4.1 Large needle driver

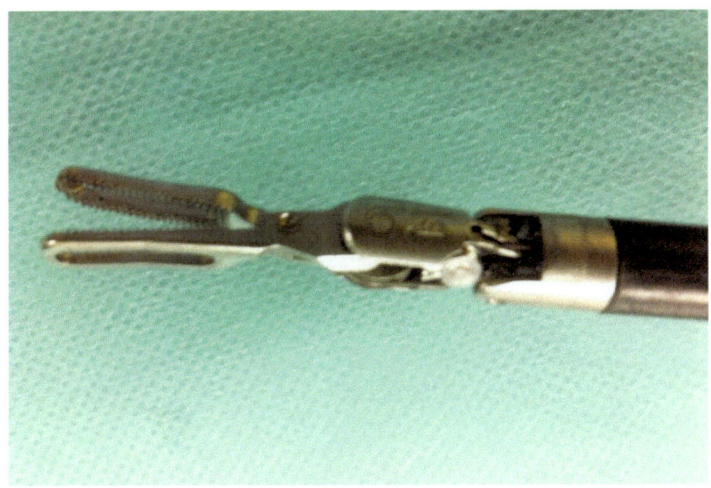

FIGURE 4.2 Prograsp™ forceps

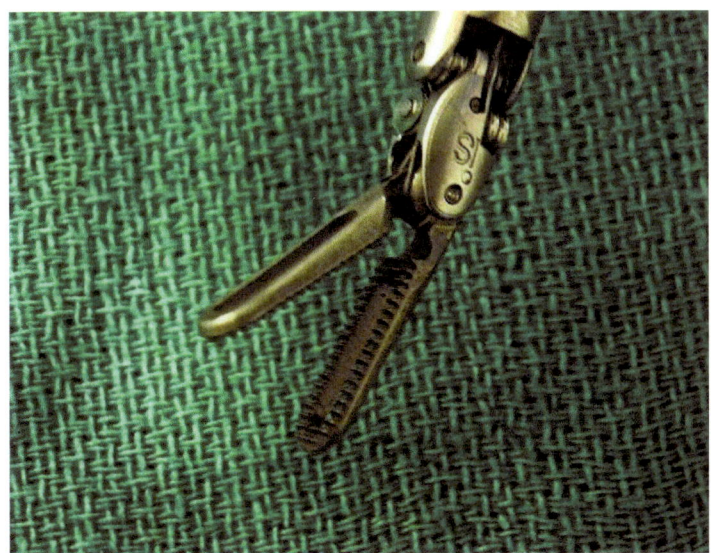

FIGURE 4.3 Cadiere forceps (preferably used in prostatectomy)

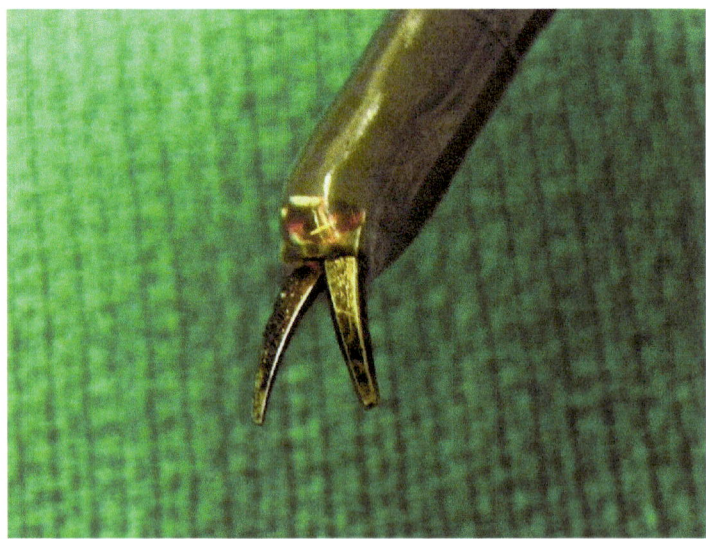

Figure 4.4 Hot Shears™ (monopolar curved scissors)

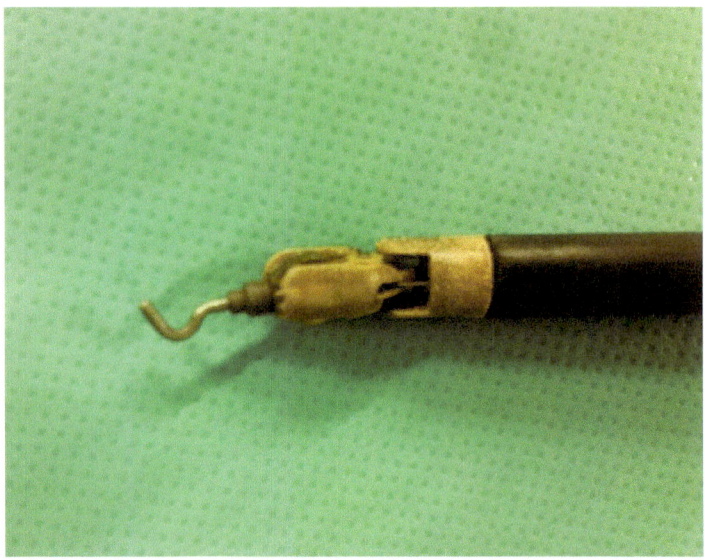

Figure 4.5 Permanent cautery hook

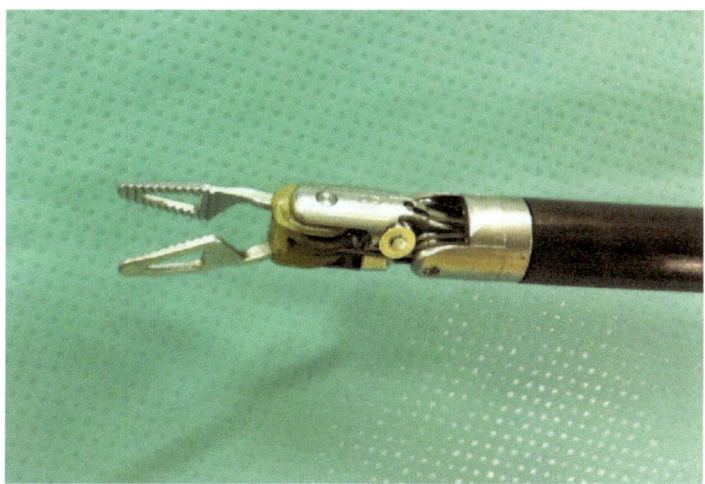

FIGURE 4.6 PreCise™ bipolar forceps

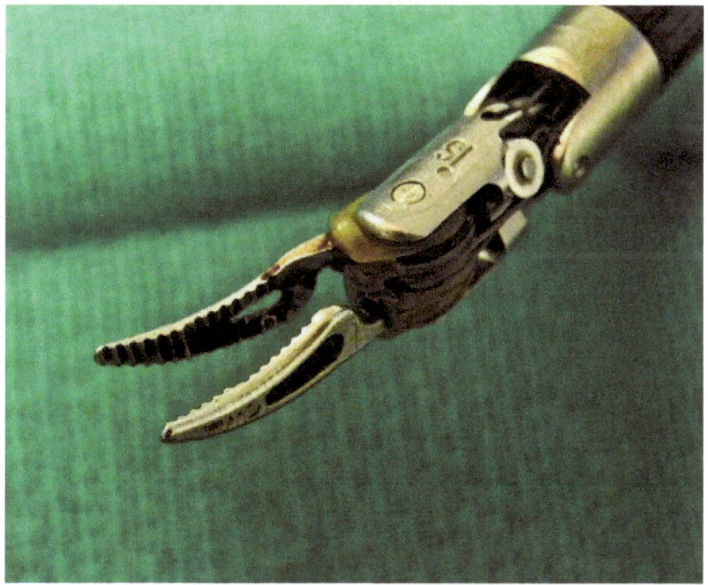

FIGURE 4.7 Maryland bipolar forceps (curved, used for prostatectomy)

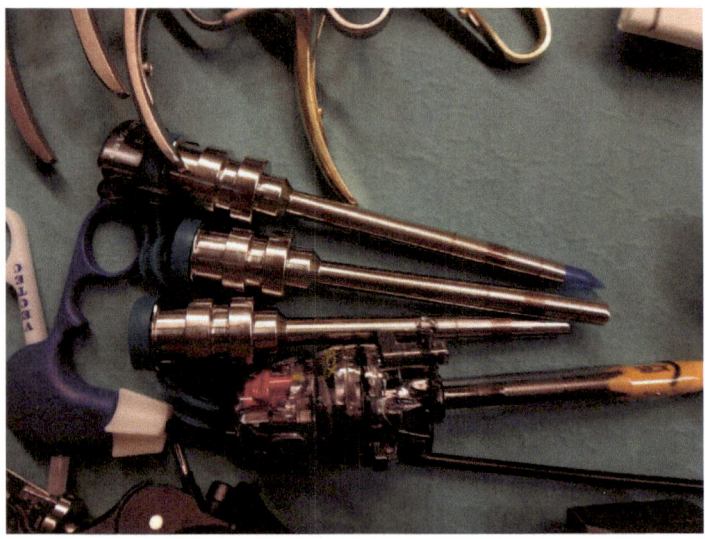

FIGURE 4.8 Cannulas, obturators and seals

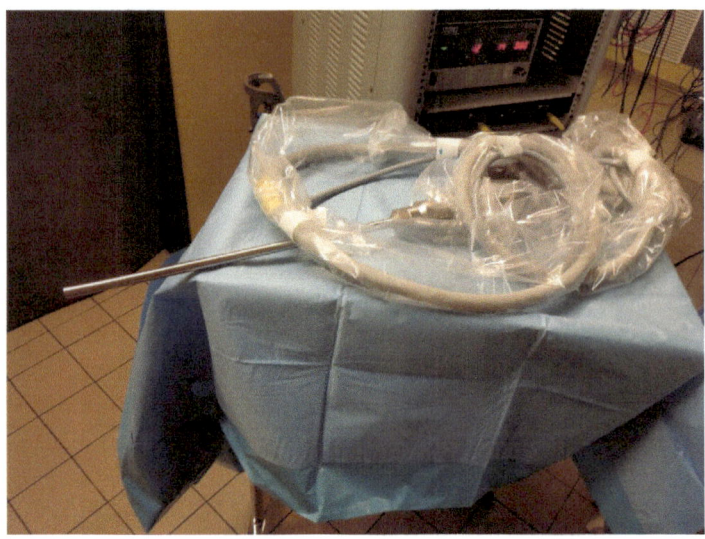

FIGURE 4.9 Camera and 0° endoscope

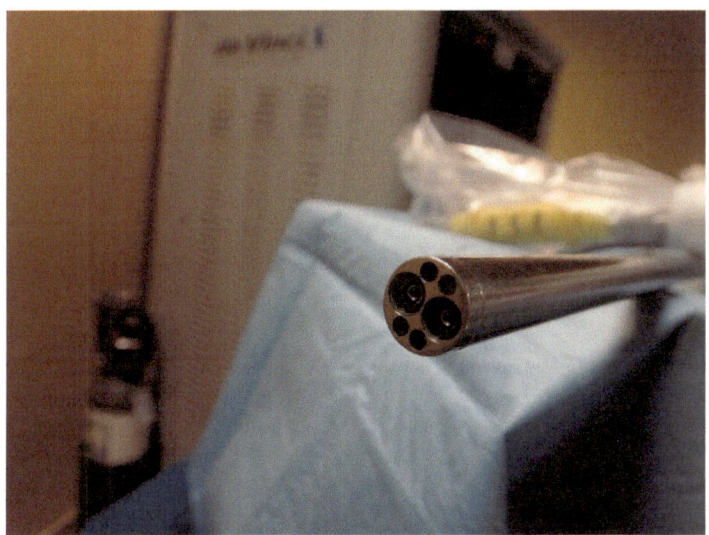

FIGURE 4.10 Details of the 3-D camera

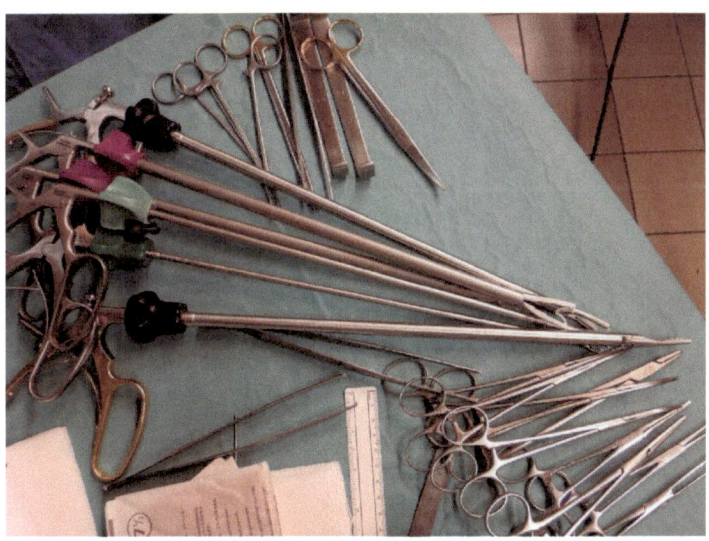

FIGURE 4.11 Manual Hem-o-lok® clips appliers

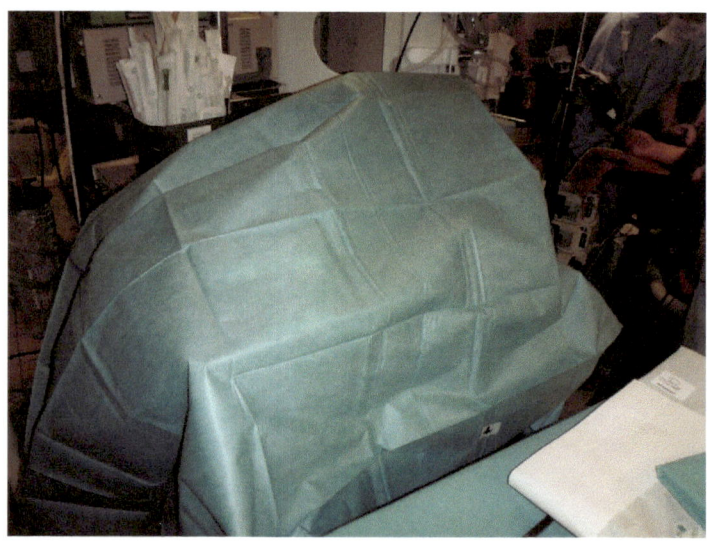

FIGURE 4.12 Laparotomy conversion table

Chapter 5
Surgical Steps

Said Abdallah Al-Mamari and Hervé Quintens

5.1 Patient Positioning

This has already been described in the Anesthesia chapter. It is important to reemphasize that like all surgical operations, final positioning must be done in the presence of both the Surgeon and the Anesthetist once the patient has been fully anesthetized, intubated and ventilated. During all previous maneuvers, the patient-side robotic cart is kept at a good distance from the patient (possibly in a corner) and protected with a sterile drape from inadvertent contact with the circulating staff (Fig. 5.1).

5.2 Skin Disinfection

The patient's skin is disinfected with a betadine® solution from the Xyphoid level to the thighs, and up to posterior axillary lines on both sides. This is done twice; first by the circulating nurse, then by the instrumentist or the assistant-surgeon

S.A. Al-Mamari (✉)
Department of Urology, The Royal Hospital,
Muscat, Oman
e-mail: sabdal67@yahoo.com

H. Quintens
Department of Urology, L'Archet 2 Hospital,
University Hospital of Nice, Nice, France

S.A. Al-Mamari, H. Quintens (eds.), *Robotic Donor Nephrectomy*, DOI 10.1007/978-3-319-04588-7_5,
© Springer International Publishing Switzerland 2014

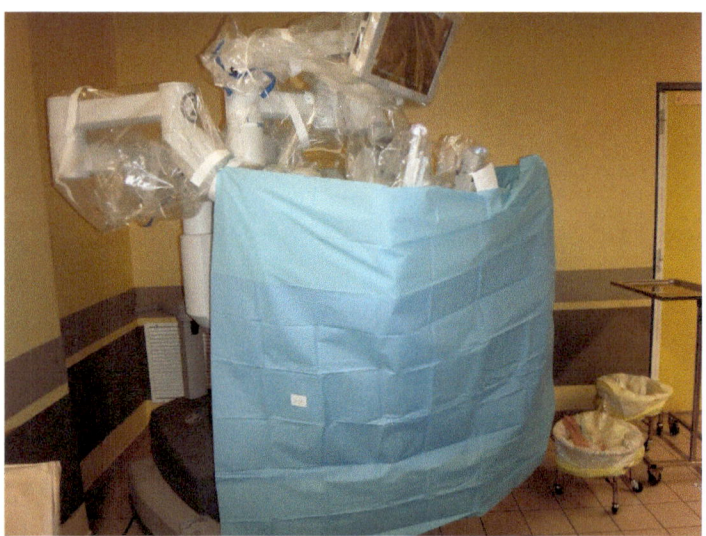

FIGURE 5.1 The robotic cart protected with a sterile drape

(Fig. 5.2). A four-piece sterile drape is used to circumscribe a large rectangular abdominal space limited by the mid-axillary line bilaterally, superiorly and inferiorly by the xyphoid and the pubis respectively (Fig. 5.3).

5.3   Pneumoperitoneum Creation, Laparoscopic Ports Placement, and Robotic Arms Docking

As for all laparoscopic procedures, the equipment check is capital before the operation starts. Apart from ensuring all robotic instruments are functioning and the camera is well calibrated, attention is paid to the carbon dioxide tanks. A second spare must be available in the OT room.

The first surgical steps are the same as for all laparoscopic renal surgeries. The summary presented below is given as a general guidance and must be adapted according to the patient's

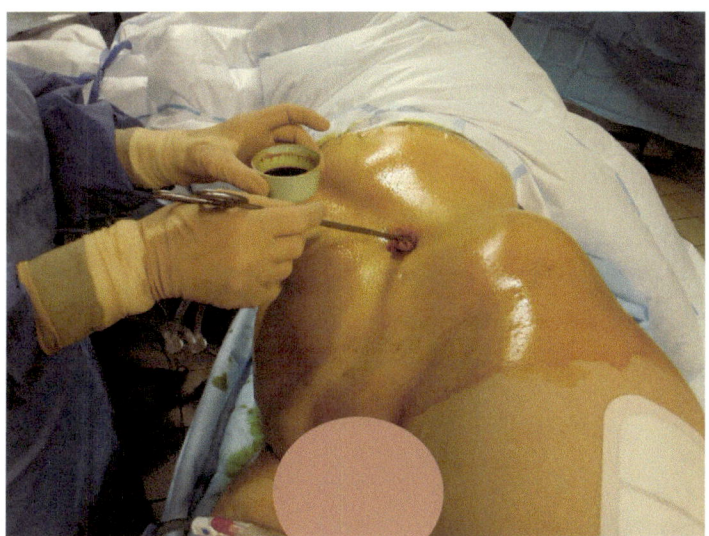

FIGURE 5.2 Skin disinfection with betadine solution

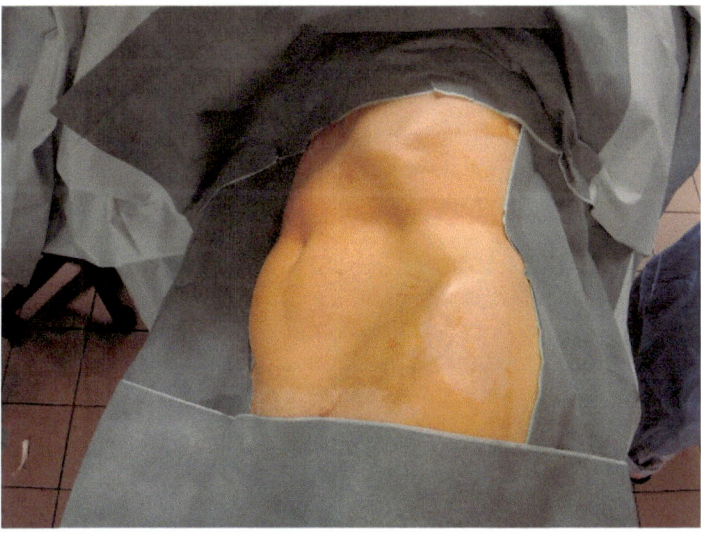

FIGURE 5.3 Patient covered with sterile drapes leaving a large abdominal access which includes the Pfannenstiel area

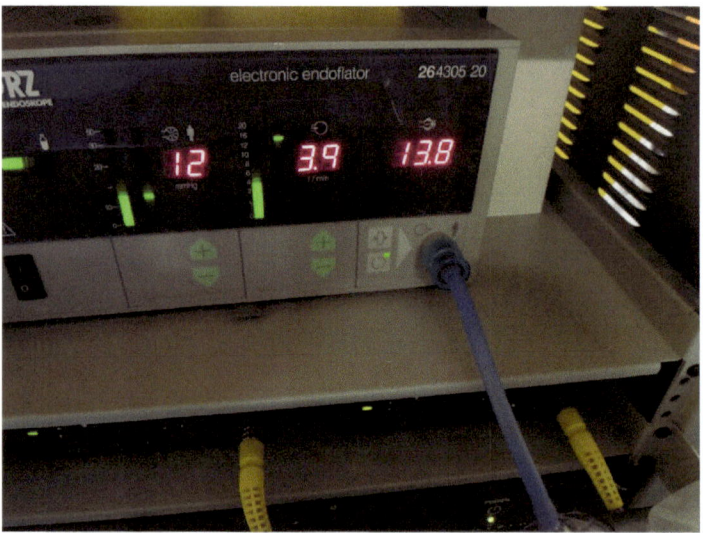

FIGURE 5.4 Peritoneal pressure monitor

body habitus since this can affect the placement of the ports: the initial ports may need to be adjusted when the patient has a history of past abdominal surgery in order to address the problem of expected adhesions; all the ports are better moved laterally in obese and superiorly in very tall patients to facilitate lateral and superior perinephric dissection [1].

We recommend the open Hasson technique because of its safety.

For the left side nephrectomy, the first 12 mm-port is created at the intersection between the left pararectal line and an oblique line between the umbilicus and the lowest level of the ribcage. Once the peritoneum cavity access is confirmed, the pneumoperitoneum is created and pressure parameters monitored (Fig. 5.4). The camera is introduced to visualize cannulas introduced from the next ports. These are created in the following order (Fig. 5.5):

• a 10-mm port four finger-breadths in an oblique line from the first port to the iliac crest, for the monopolar scissor or the permanent cautery hook (this can be inverted with the next port for left-handed surgeons),

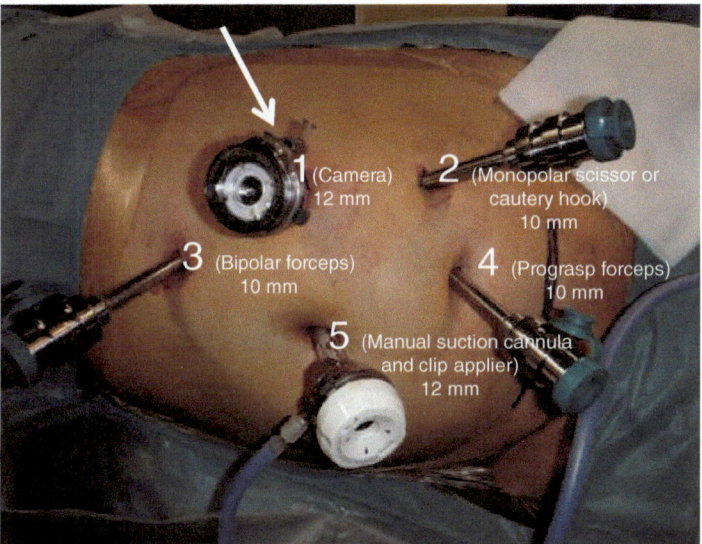

1 (Camera) 12 mm

2 (Monopolar scissor or cautery hook) 10 mm

3 (Bipolar forceps) 10 mm

4 (Prograsp forceps) 10 mm

5 (Manual suction cannula and clip applier) 12 mm

FIGURE 5.5 Laparoscopic ports sites and robotic cannulas in position: the numbers indicate the chronology of ports creation as well as the corresponding robotic arm to be docked (up to number *4*). The instruments to be used through each port are mentioned between brackets and the port sizes are given below. The *arrow* indicates the oblique axis of the robotic cart in the direction of the camera port and perpendicular to the line between ports *2* and *3*

- a 10-mm port four finger-breadths in sub-costal position at a vertical line from the first port to the rib cage, for the bipolar forceps,
- a 10-mm port four finger-breadths from the second port in the pararectal line at the level of the anterior superior iliac spine, for the prograsp forceps,
- a 12-mm port at the umbilicus for the manual suction device and the clip-applier to be controlled by the assistant. It helps also for the introduction of compresses, sutures, manual scissors, etc.…

Once all five ports are created, the patient's side robotic cart is **obliquely** advanced to the patient aiming the camera port in an axis perpendicular to the line between the second and the third ports through which the two most deployed instruments will be used (Figs. 5.5 and 5.6a, b).

The four robotic arms are docked to the cannulas (Fig. 5.7), the instruments are mounted on the robotic arms, the cautery tools are connected to the electro-surgical unit, and the cutting and coagulation values are adjusted according to the Surgeon's preference (Fig. 5.8).

However it is important to note that experienced Surgeons tend to use only three arms: one for the camera and two for the operating tools (the monopolar scissor or the permanent cautery hook being controlled by the dominant hand, and bipolar forceps by the other hand). This strategy is guided by financial reasons and is particularly feasible in non-obese patients.

Figures 5.9 and 5.10 show the operation site after instruments docking and a whole view of the operating theater when the complete set-up is ready.

For the right nephrectomy, patient's positioning is mutatis mutandis the same as abovementioned: the patient lies now in a left semi-lateral position with the back turned to the robot cart. The laparoscopic ports' topography is:

- a 12-mm port in the right pararectal line at the horizontal level of the umbilicus for the camera (1st robotic arm),
- a 10-mm port in the right pararectal line 1–2 cm below the ribcage for the monopolar scissor or the cautery hook (second robotic arm),
- a 10-mm port 1–2 cm above and medial to the right antero-superior iliac spine for the Bipolar Precise® Grasper (third robotic arm),
- a 12-mm port at the umbilicus for the assistant suction device and clip-appliers,
- a 5-mm is inserted in the midline at the level of the second port for the liver retractor,
- if required, a 10-mm port is created in the right pararectal line just above the iliac crest for the fourth robotic arm.

For the sake of clarity, we will initially describe the technical aspects of the left donor nephrectomy, then we will address the particular points of the right side donor nephrectomy, and at the end we will comment on the final common steps.

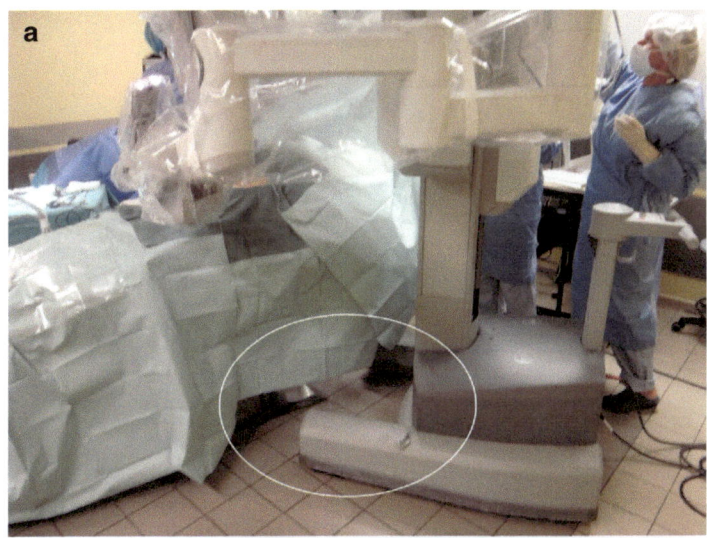

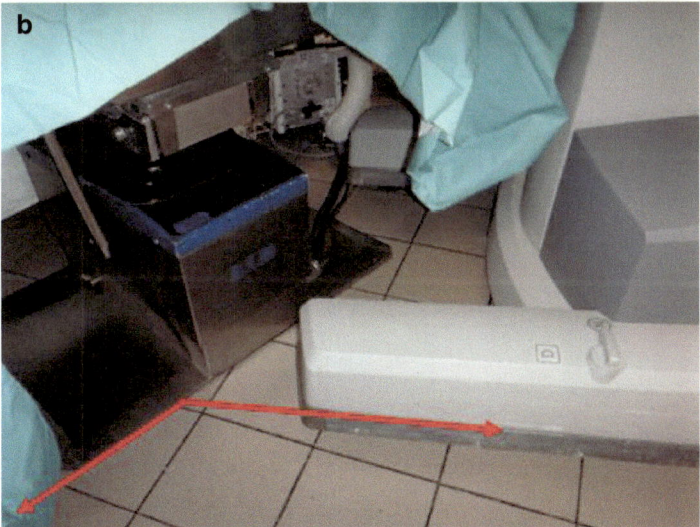

FIGURE 5.6 (**a**) Oblique approach of the robotic cart at the patient's left shoulder for a left nephrectomy (see the *circle* and the Fig. 5.6b). (**b**) Angle formed by the robot cart foot and the operating table

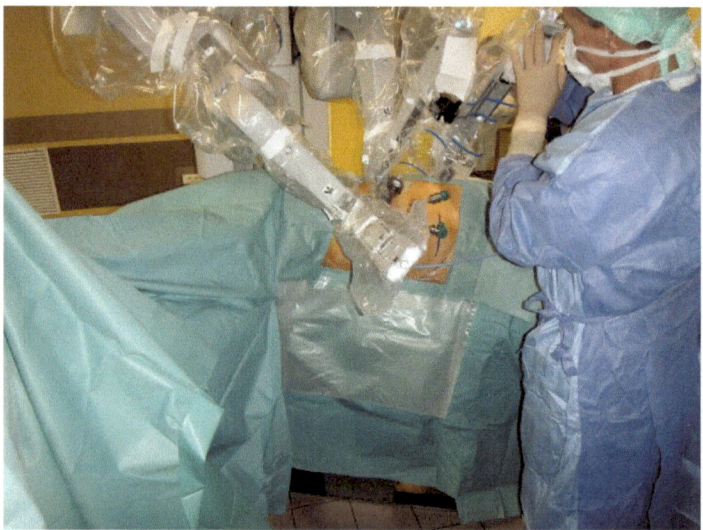

FIGURE 5.7 Docking of the robotic instruments

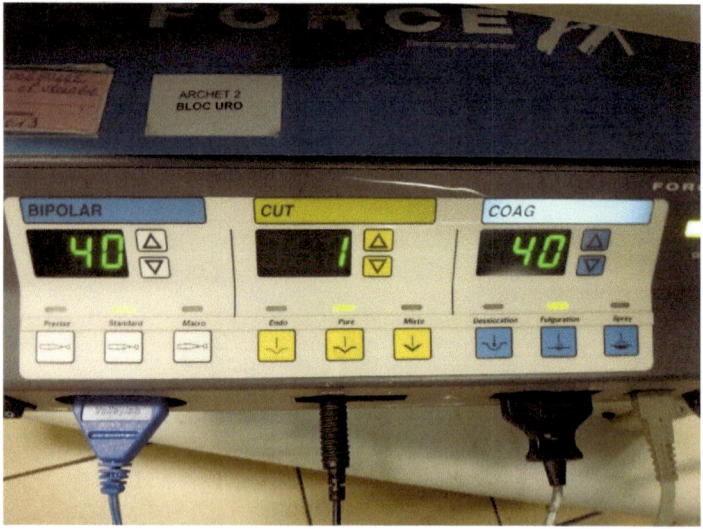

FIGURE 5.8 Electrosurgical unit

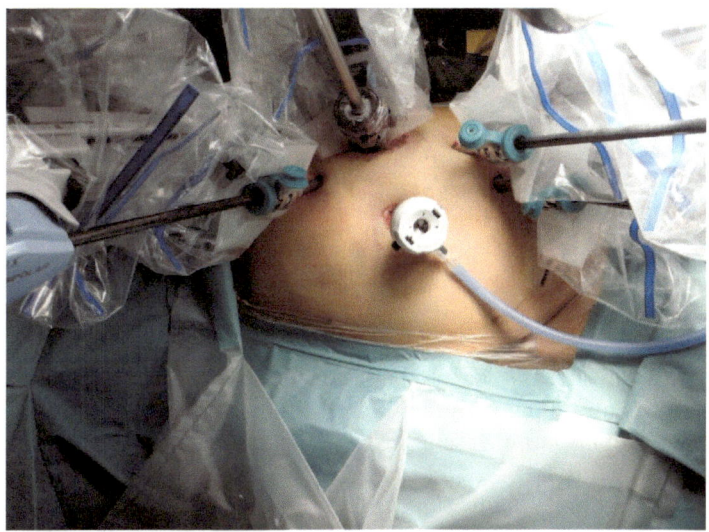

FIGURE 5.9 View of the ports and instruments after docking

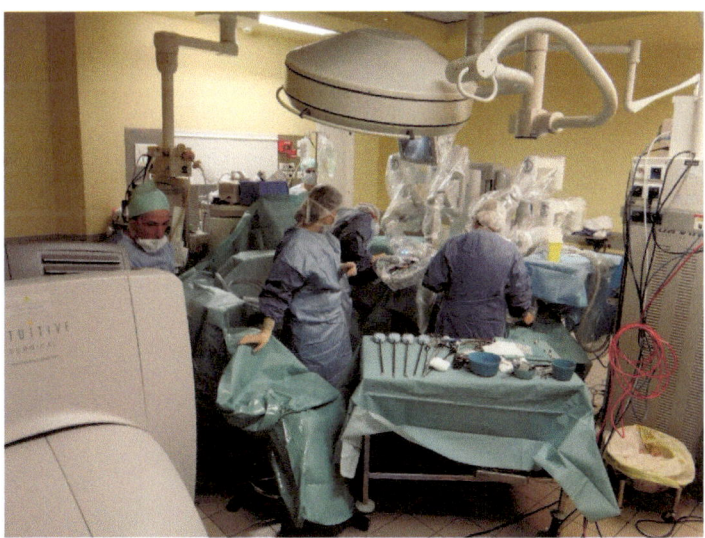

FIGURE 5.10 The set-up is completed. Now the Surgeon will seat in front of the console and start the telemanipulation of the robotic cart

5.4   Left Donor Nephrectomy

Generally the procedure starts with the dissection of the splenic flexure of the colon along the avascular Toldt's white line. However if intra-peritoneal adhesions are present, these will be dealt with first (Fig. 5.11).

The fascia of Toldt is incised to free the left colic angle from the abdominal wall in order to access the retroperitoneal space (Fig. 5.12a, b). Then the phreno-colic, splenocolic and spleno-renal ligaments are divided (Fig. 5.13). This allows the upper pole of the kidney with its covering Gerota's fascia to be seen. Dissection is followed downwards along the white line of Toldt through a plane between the Zuckerkandl fascia posteriorly and the mesocolon anteriorly until the left colon falls medially with its attached peritoneum. At this time the kidney with its covering fascia is left attached to the posterior abdominal wall (Fig. 5.14). The dissection of the fascia of Toldt is continued caudally (Fig. 5.15). The retroperitoneal space is entered and fatty

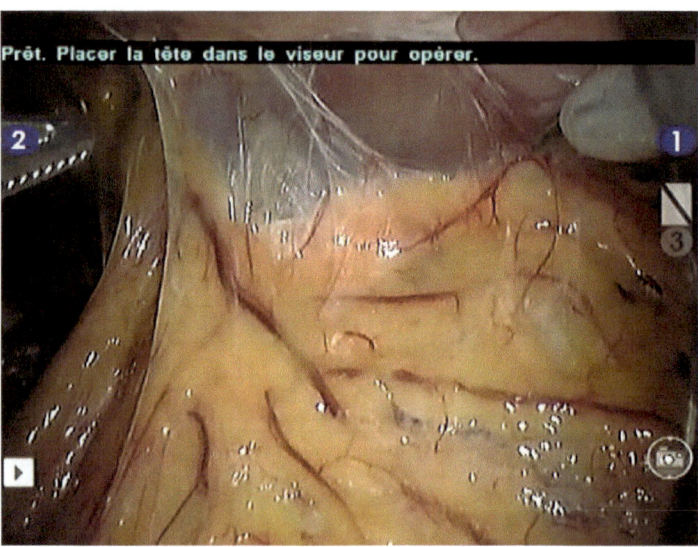

FIGURE 5.11 Intra-peritoneal adhesions being released

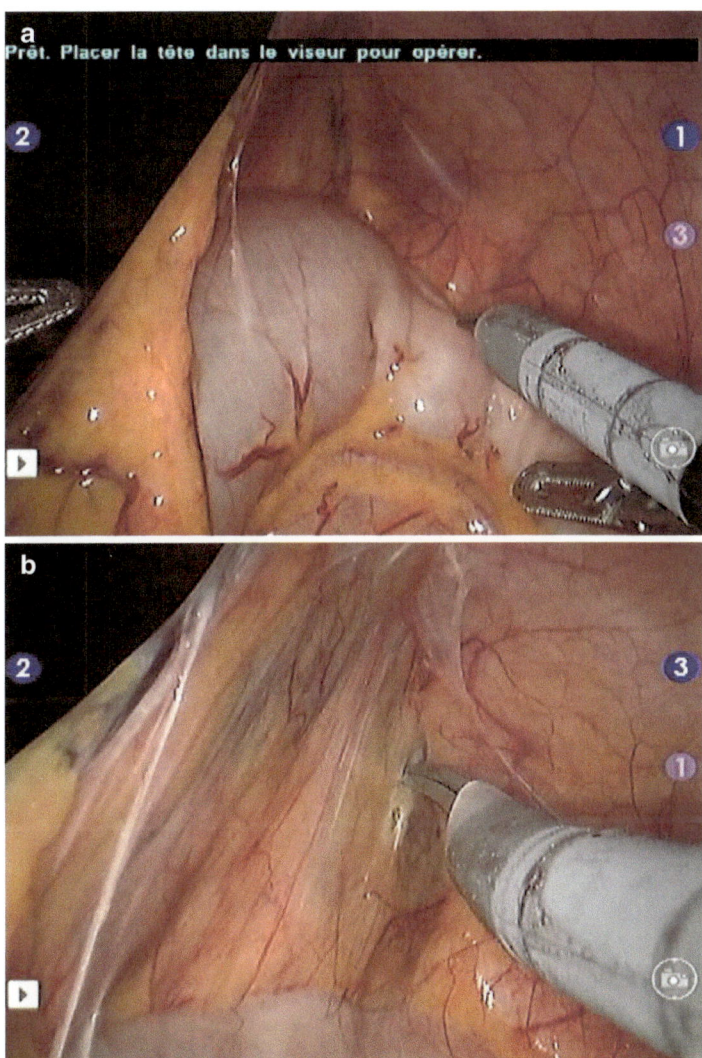

FIGURE 5.12 (a) View of the left colic angle and the fascia of Toldt. (b) The fascia of Toldt is dissected using a cautery scissor, to free the left colic angle from the abdominal wall

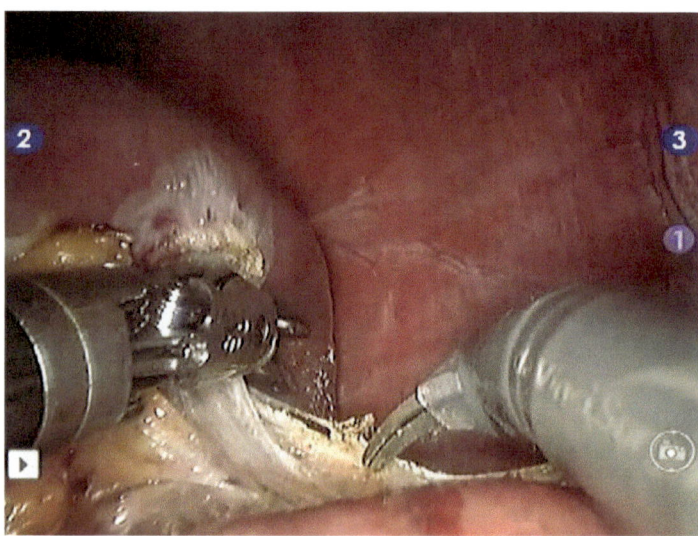

FIGURE 5.13 Division of the spleno-renal ligament

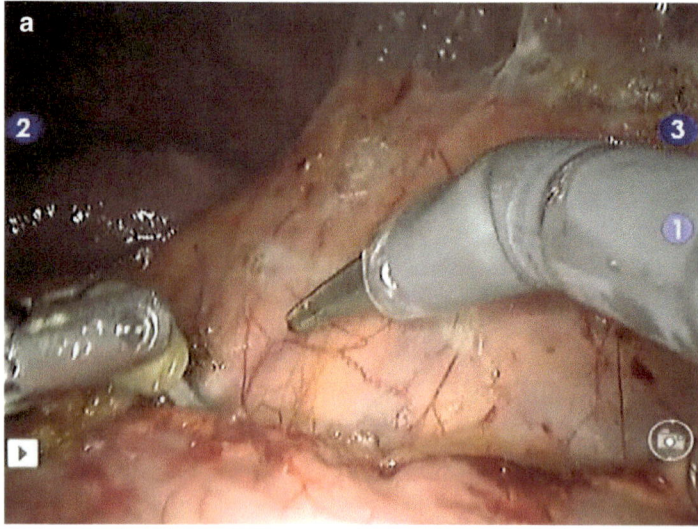

FIGURE 5.14 (**a**) Dissection along the white line of Toldt. (**b**) The left colic angle has fallen medially revealing the fatty fascia covering the kidney with its covering fatty fascia

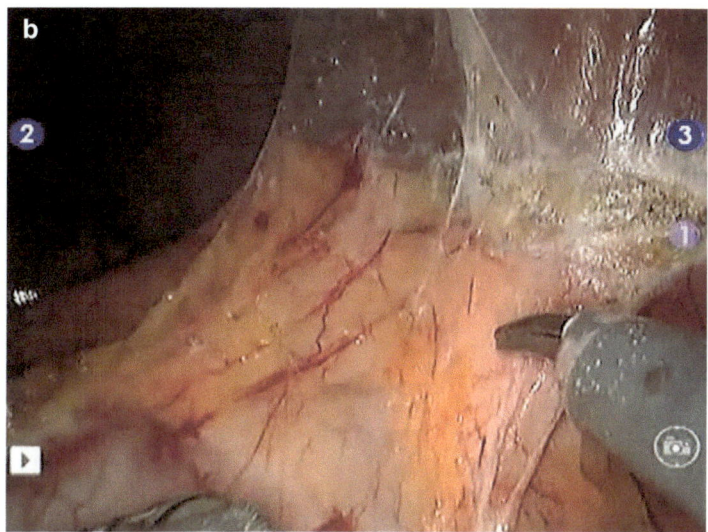

FIGURE 5.14 (continued)

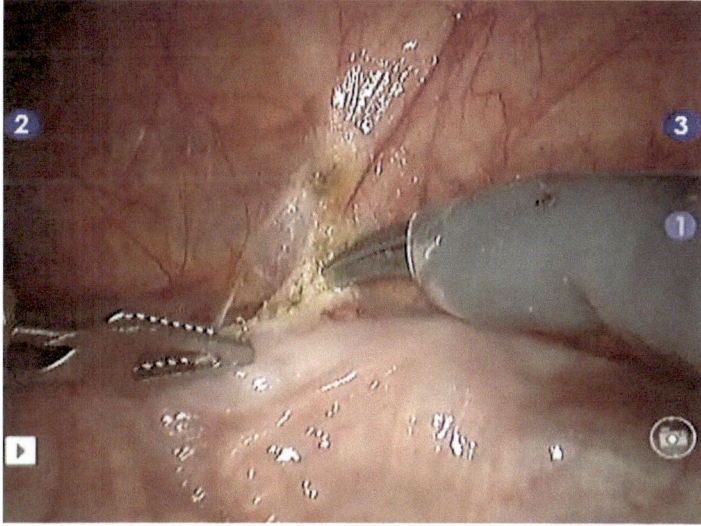

FIGURE 5.15 Dissection of the white line of Toldt is continued more caudally

tissues are incised using the bipolar forceps and the monopolar scissor (or the cautery hook) until the left gonadal
vein is reached. This is then freed from its posterior attachments and the psoas muscle is displayed (Fig. 5.16a, b). At
this level, the ureter is seen medial to the gonadal vein. It is
delicately held by its surrounding fascia and its loose posterior attachments are released up to the psoas muscle
(Fig. 5.17a, b). Now the gonadal vein is followed cranially
where it crosses the ureter and lies medial to it. Dissection
is continued until the left renal vein is reached and its anterior aspect dissected. The characteristic venous violet cross
appears; it is formed by the confluences of the adrenal and
gonadal veins into the left renal vein (Fig. 5.18). At this step,
the assistant retracts the medial lip of the opened Gerota's
fatty fascia with the aid of a compress held by the suction
cannula (Fig. 5.19). This maneuver allows a better exposure
and dissection of the adrenal vein which is clipped with two
Hem-o-loks distally and one proximally, and sectioned by
the robotic scissor (Fig. 5.20a, b). The Prograsp forceps
docked to the robot's fourth arm holds the lateral lip of the
Gerota's fascia and lifts the kidney up. This allows a good
exposure of the gonadal vein which is clipped and sectioned
to allow dissection of the posterior aspect of the left renal
vein (Fig. 5.21). If the monopolar scissor was used so far, it
is better replaced now by the cautery hook and further dissection is carried out around the renal vein. This is done
with a maximum of patience, millimeter by millimeter, until
the reno-azygo-lumbar vein is visualized on the posterior
aspect of the renal vein (Fig. 5.22). It is dissected and sectioned between two Hem-o-lok® clips (Fig. 5.23). Now the
renal vein is free all around. Again the cautery hook
replaces the monopolar scissor and hilar dissection is performed further posteriorly (Fig. 5.24). The renal artery is
soon seen after some fatty tissues have been cleared. When
two arteries are present as shown in our selected case, the
first artery is seen and dissected all around, then the second
(Fig. 5.25a, b). The forthcoming steps are similar to the right
side donor nephrectomy and are dealt with in paragraph 6.

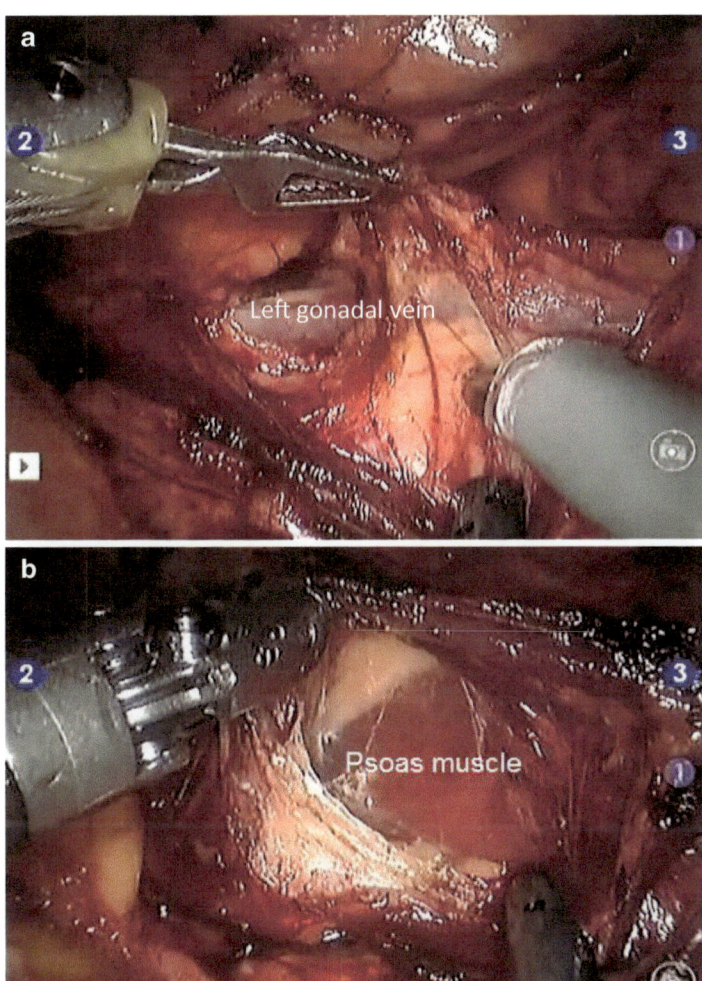

FIGURE 5.16 (**a**) View of the left gonadal vein freed of fatty tissue (note the action of the PreCise™ Bipolar Forceps lifting the vein by catching on its covering fatty fascia, with the monopolar scissor cutting its posterior attachments while the sucking cannula aspirates smoke and retracts the colon). (**b**) The gonadal vein is lifted by the bipolar forceps and the psoas muscle is displayed

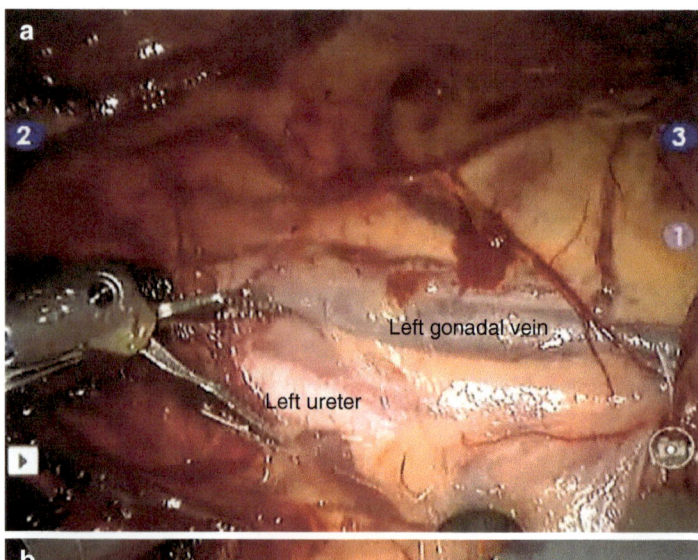

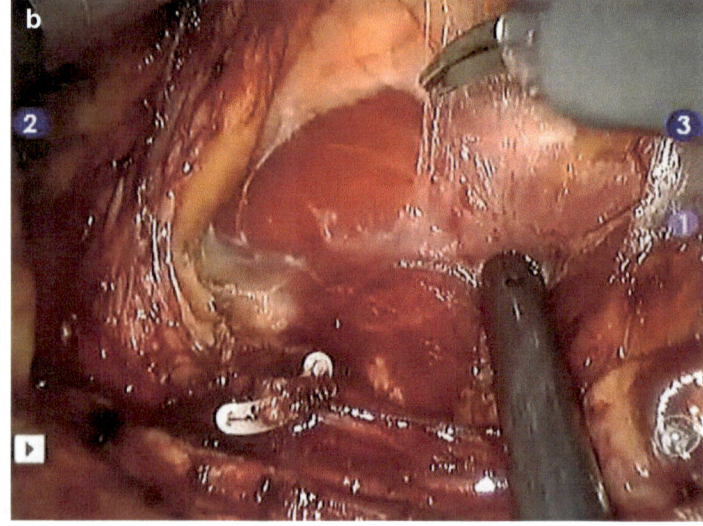

FIGURE 5.17 (**a**) View of the left ureter and gonadal vein. At this level the ureter is seen medial to the gonadal vein. Few centimeters above, the vein will cross in front of the ureter to lie medially. (**b**) Both the ureter and the gonadal vein are lifted and their loose posterior attachments to the psoas muscle are released with the monopolar scissor

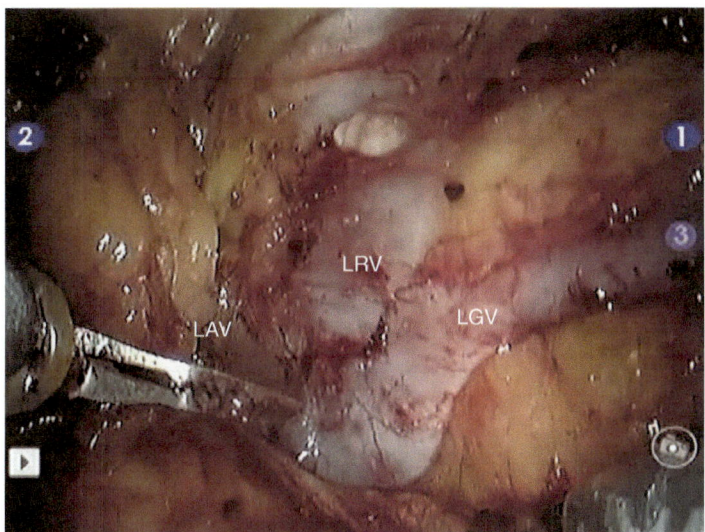

FIGURE 5.18 View of the "violet cross of the left nephrectomy". *LRV* left renal vein, *LAV* left adrenal vein, *LGV* left gonadal vein

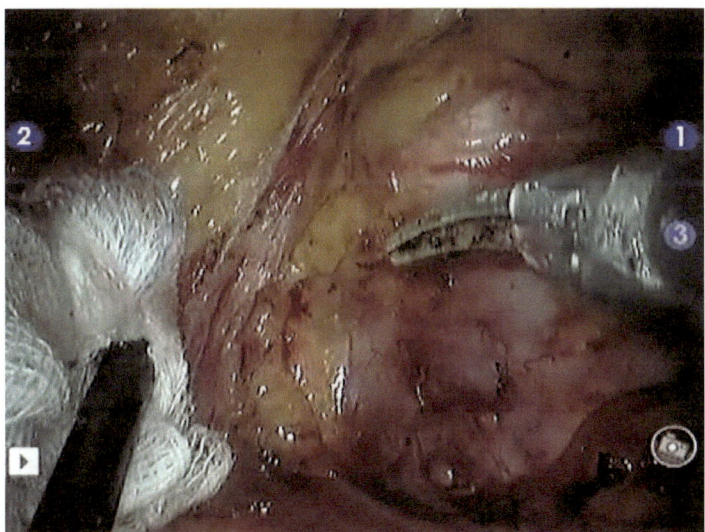

FIGURE 5.19 The assistant retracts the medial lip of the opened Gerota's fascia with the aid of a compress held by the sucking cannula

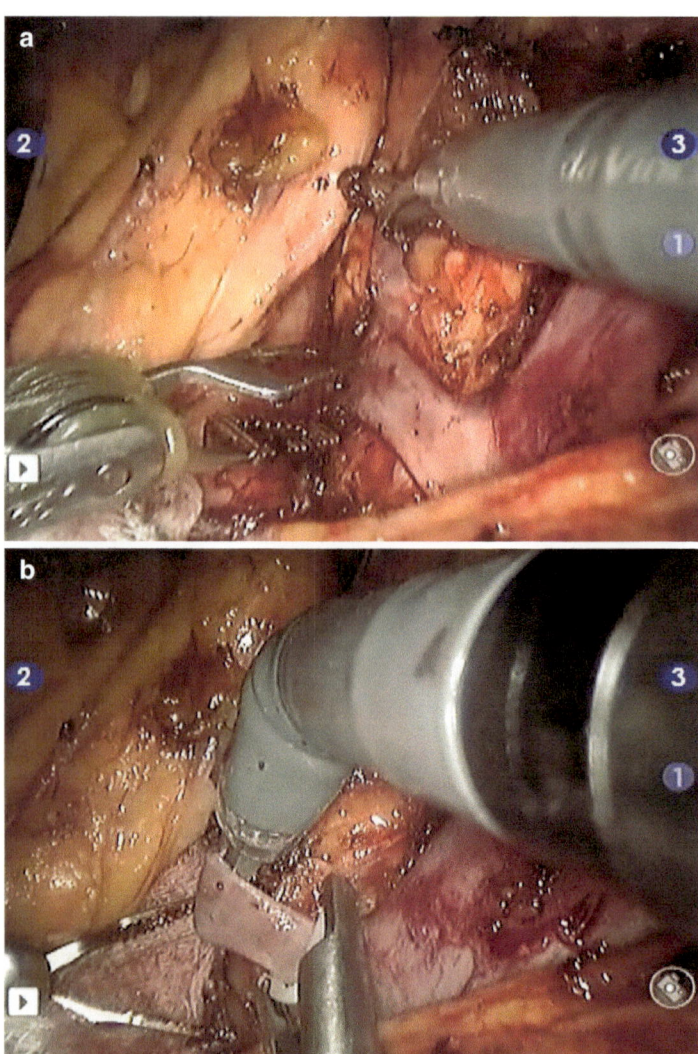

FIGURE 5.20 (**a**) Exposure of the left adrenal vein. (**b**) Clipping of the left adrenal vein. Note the action of the monopolar scissor lifting the vein to allow its optimal clipping without catching the posterior fatty tissue

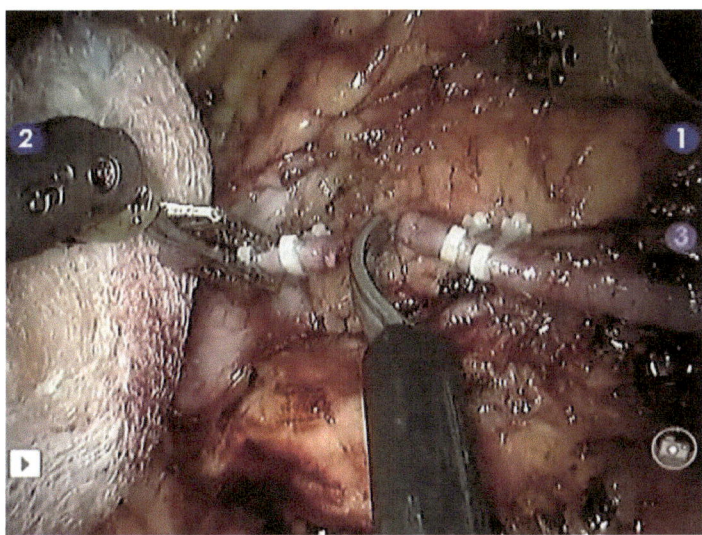

FIGURE 5.21 The gonadal vein is divided between hem-o-lock® clips. See the action of the Prograsp forceps docked to the robot's fourth arm holding the lateral lip of the Gerota's fascia and lifting the kidney up

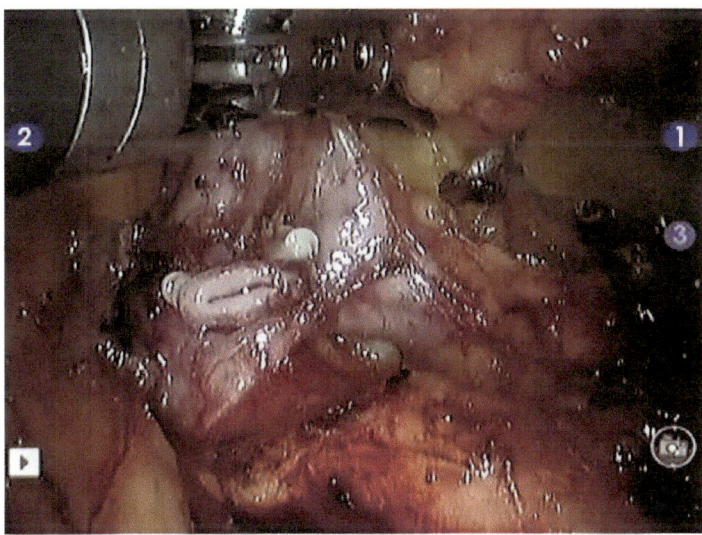

FIGURE 5.22 The reno-azygo-lumbar vein is seen on the posterior aspect of the left renal vein

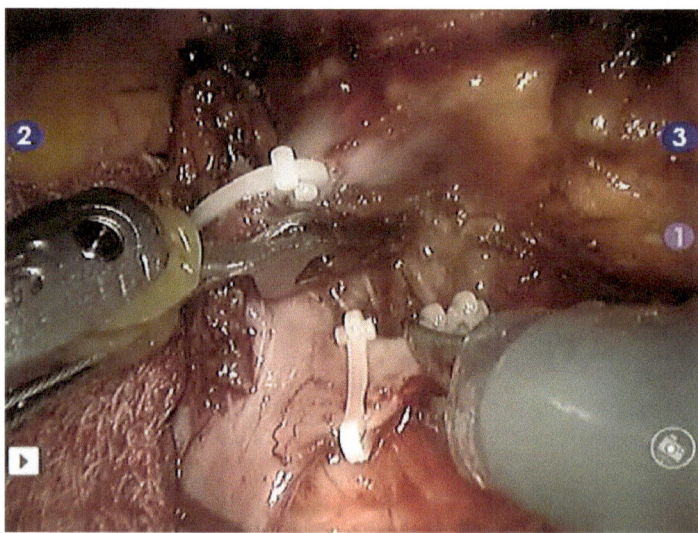

FIGURE 5.23 Division of the reno-azygo-lumbar vein between Hem-O-Locks

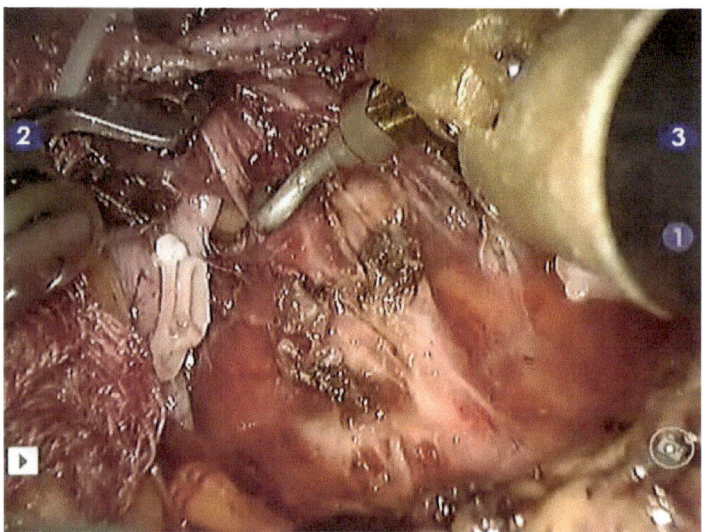

FIGURE 5.24 Dissection of the hilum carried out with the cautery hook with extreme care

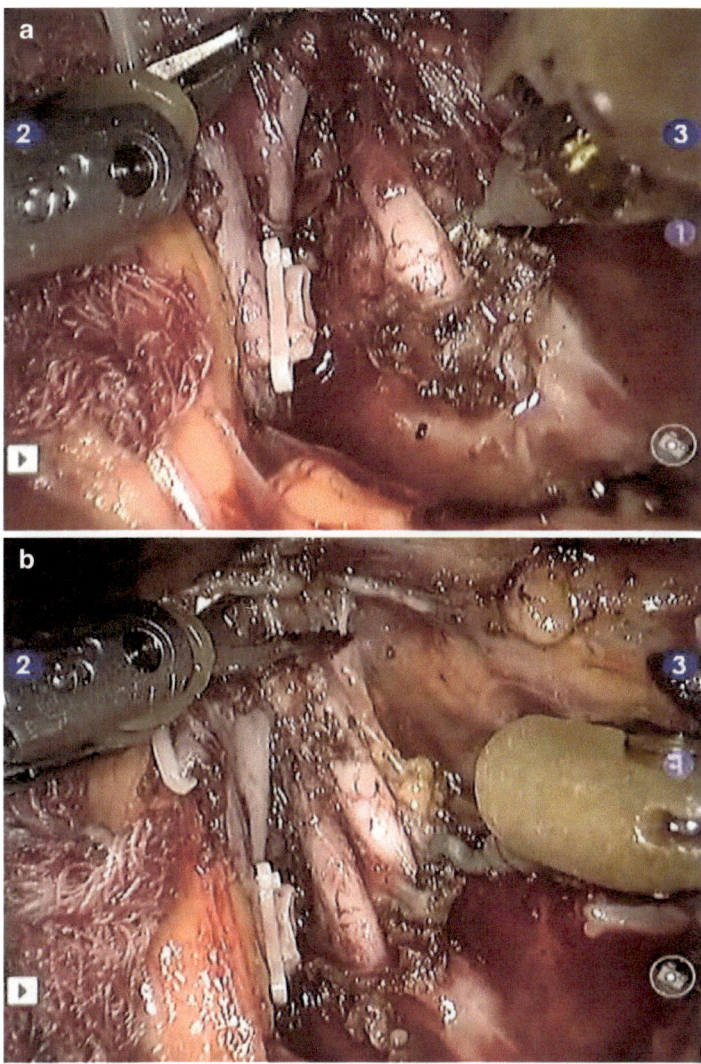

FIGURE 5.25 (**a**) View of the first renal artery posterior to the vein. (**b**) View of both left renal arteries

5.5   Right Donor Nephrectomy

Right side donor nephrectomy is estimated to occur in about 10–15 % of all donor nephrectomies [2], the left kidney being preferred for its longer vein which allows an easier anastomosis in the recipient site. However there are few indications which necessitate a right side nephrectomy. These include the presence of multiple arteries on the left side which would complicate the transplantation technique and a suboptimal right kidney split function (e.g. with a value around 40 %) which may expose the healthy donor to the risk of renal function impairment after left nephrectomy.

The first step involves incision of the avascular white line of Toldt to free the right colic angle and to reach the Gerota's fascia which is not opened at this point to allow the colon to fall medially (Figs. 5.26 and 5.27).

Once the colon has fallen medially, a liver retractor is inserted and fixed to the abdominal wall (Fig. 5.28). Further

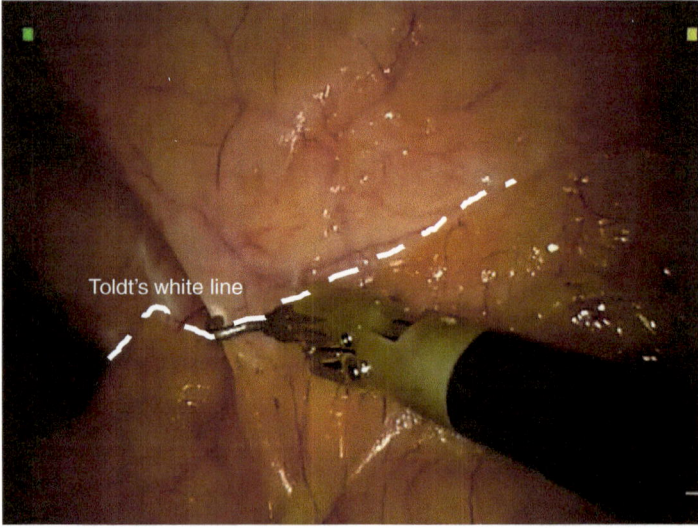

FIGURE 5.26 Right colic angle dissection through Toldt's line (here using a cautery hook)

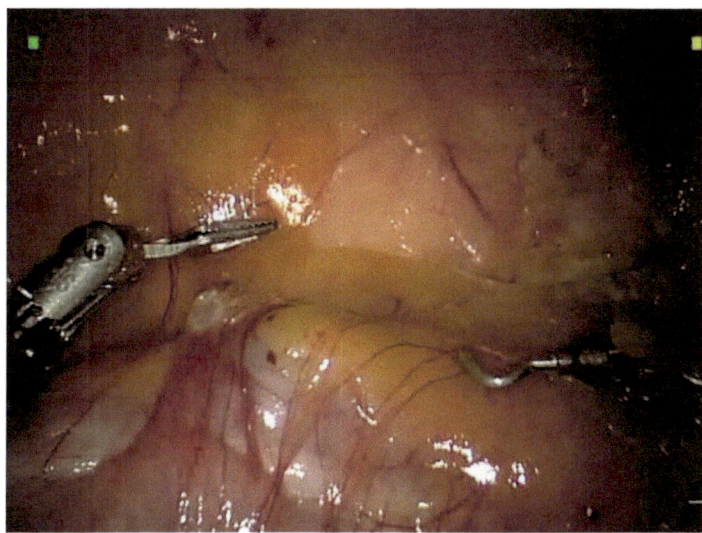

FIGURE 5.27 The colon is falling medially revealing a "fatty mount": this is the Gerota's fascia covering the underlining right kidney and adrenal gland

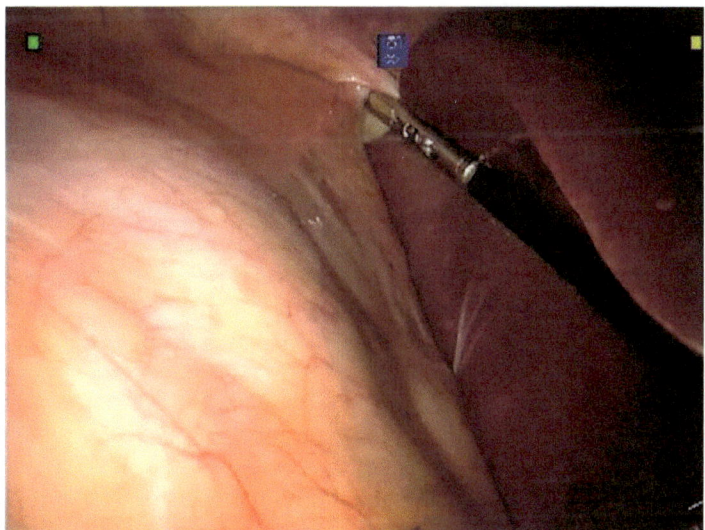

FIGURE 5.28 A retractor catching the abdominal wall to lift the liver

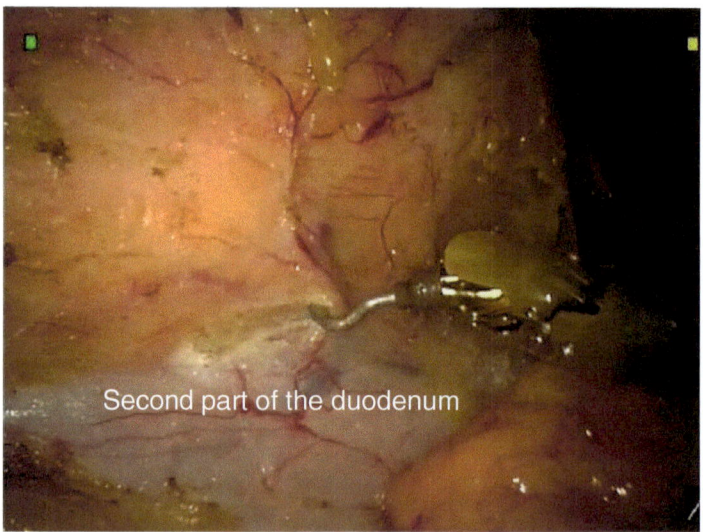

Second part of the duodenum

FIGURE 5.29 Hook dissection at the base of the fatty Gerota's fascia just lateral to the Second part of the duodenum

dissection using the cautery hook is carried out lateral to the second part of the duodenum at the floor of the "fatty mount" formed by Gerota's fascia with the aim of seeing the inferior vena cava (Figs. 5.29 and 5.30). When revealed, the anterior and right lateral faces of the IVC are cleared of the covering tissue in order to reach the right renal vein confluence. Not infrequently, the dissection of the anterior face of the IVC below the renal veins level may injure the right gonadal vein. This will appear first as mild bleeding which will increase with every coagulation attempt, and will soon obscure the area (Figs. 5.31 and 5.32). It is wise here to put pressure on the bleeding site with a compress held by the suction cannula. Then dissection is done around the fatty covering of the gonadal vein to allow a Hem-o-lok® insertion distally (Fig. 5.33) and a continuous suture of 6/0 prolene® inserted around the proximal stump (Fig. 5.34). Once this incident is overcome, dissection of the perinephric fatty fascia is continued cranially at the lateral aspect of the IVC. Here some minor, but spectacular, arterial bleeding may occur and are easily controlled with coagulation

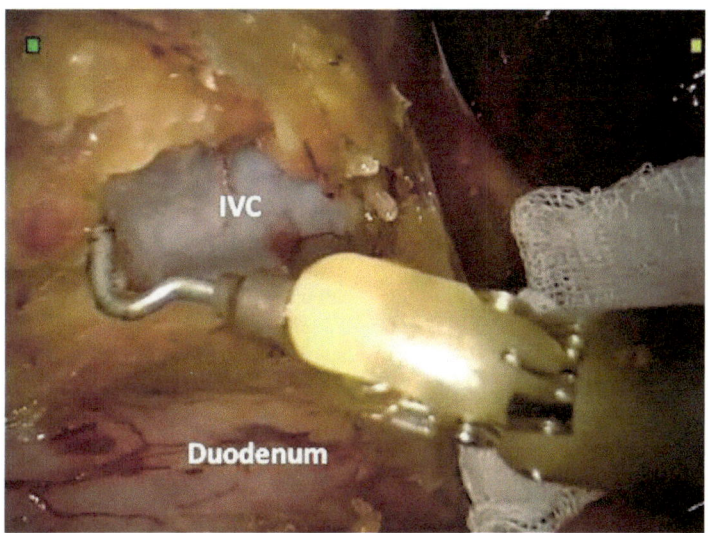

FIGURE 5.30 View of the inferior vena cava (IVC)

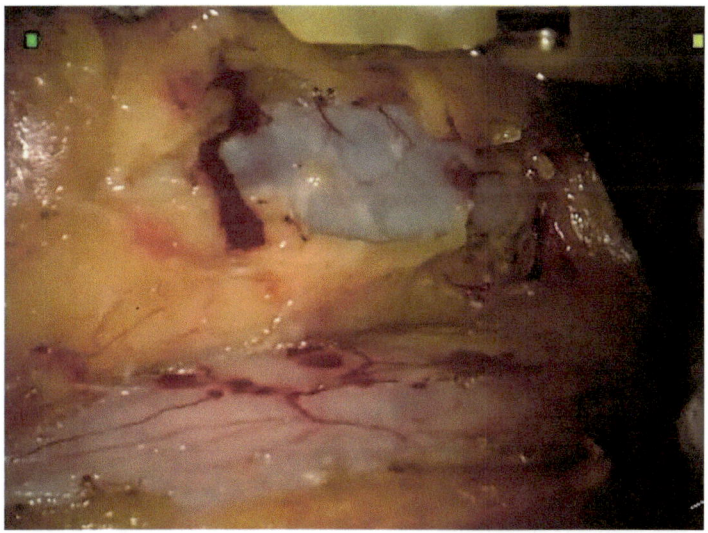

FIGURE 5.31 Beware of a right gonadal vein injury at the anterior aspect of the IVC: it will start with mild bleeding

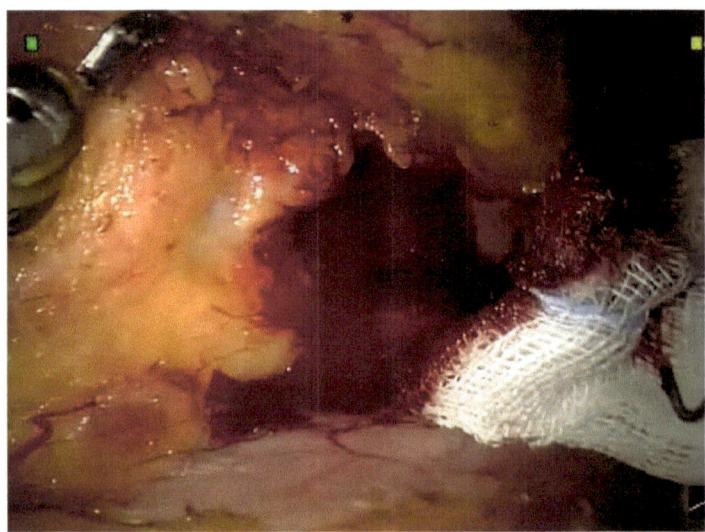

FIGURE 5.32 Rapidly obscuring right gonadal vein bleeding

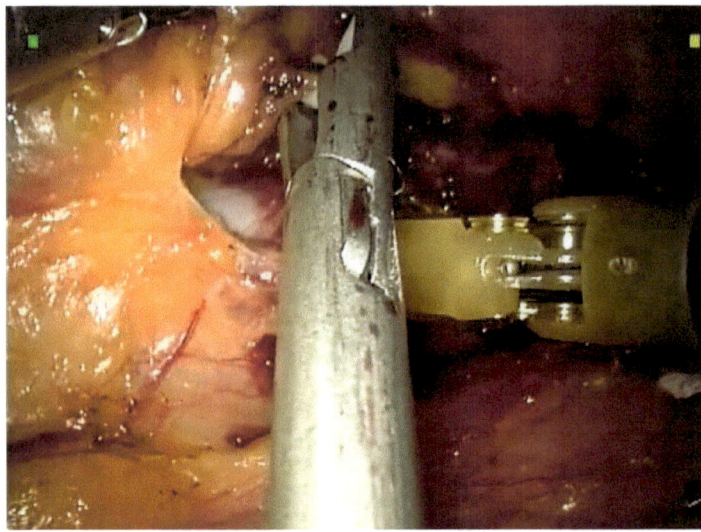

FIGUER 5.33 Clipping the gonadal vein distal to the bleeding point

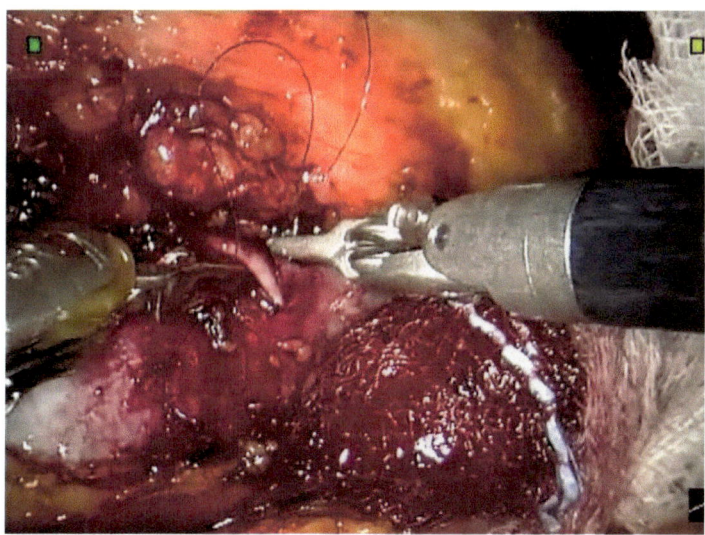

FIGURE 5.34 The gonadal vein is sutured around its insertion to the IVC

(Fig. 5.35a, b). Now the renal vein is encountered and dissected all around from its caval end toward the hilum, and it is enlaced with a rubber band which will help with its retraction (Fig. 5.36a, b). Very careful dissection is continued posteriorly to the vein with the cautery hook and the renal artery is seen and freed from the surrounding fatty tissue (Fig. 5.37). **This maneuver is continued behind the IVC up to the interaortico-caval space aiming at providing the longest artery possible for ease of the transplantation technique.**

Once the renal vessels are identified and skeletonized, the next steps are common to both right and left donor nephrectomies.

5.6   Final Common Steps

Before describing these steps, it is important to emphasize the importance of the assistant's role. More than in standard laparoscopy, he carries here greater responsibilities which are summarized into two points:

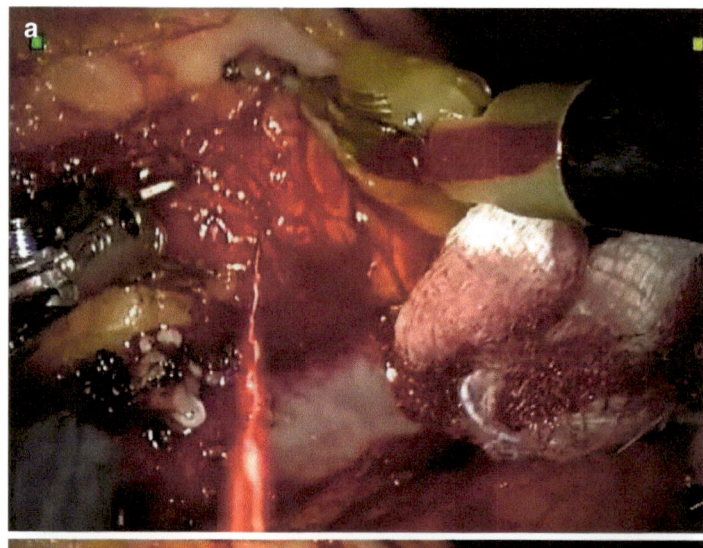

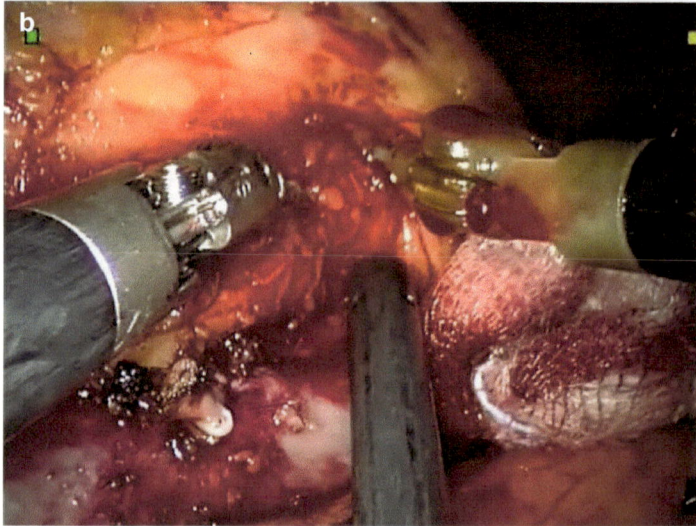

FIGURE 5.35 (**a**) The "Traffic light" of the renal hilum: spectacular arteriolar bleeding arising from the hilar fatty tissue. (**b**) The arteriolar bleeding is easily controlled with the Precise Bipolar Forceps

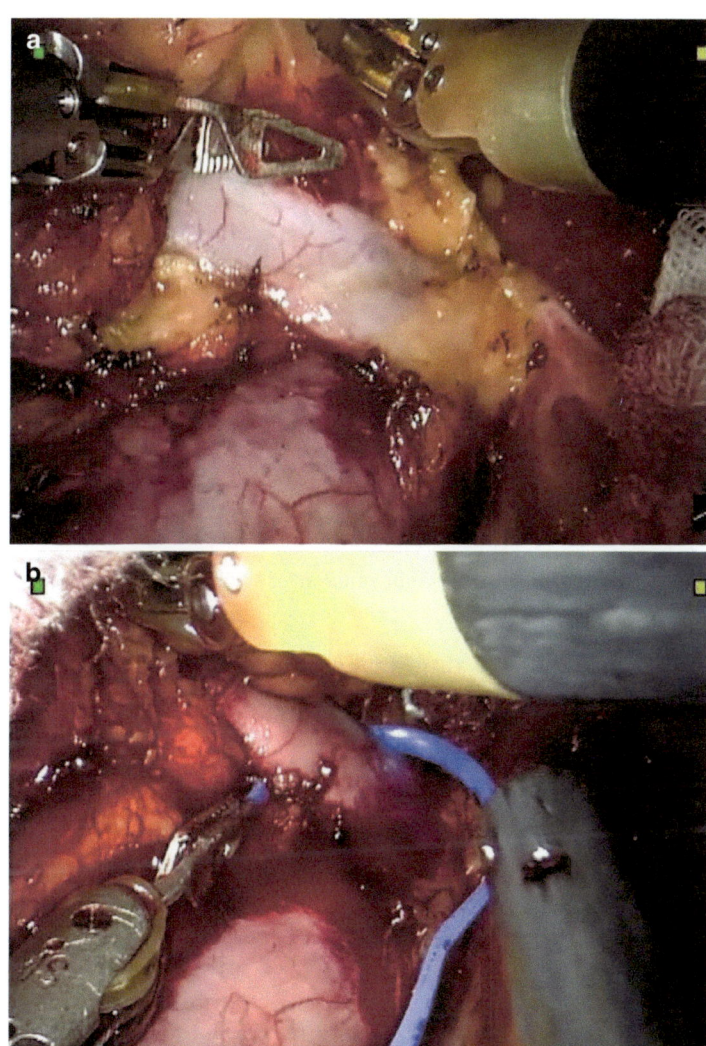

FIGURE 5.36 (**a**) View of the origin of the right renal vein. (**b**) A rubber band is used to enlace the right renal vein. It will help to retract the vein in the next steps

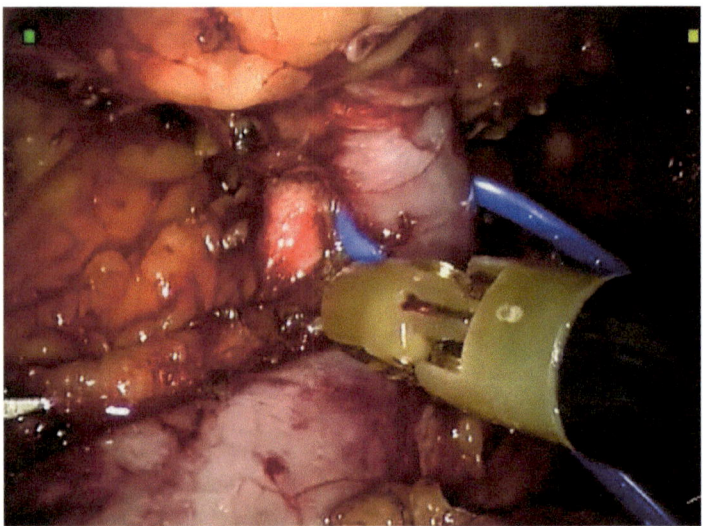

FIGURE 5.37 View of the right renal artery behind the vein

- He will perform the Pfannenstiel incision through which he will insert the Endocatch™ and will retrieve the kidney.
- Moreover, he will apply the Hem-o-lok® clips on the renal vessels, and may even be requested to divide them if only three robotic arms are used.

This is why in the current practice the assistant in robotic donor nephrectomy is generally a Senior Resident with enough experience and skill in laparoscopic surgery. The advent of new instruments such as the Endowrist® Clip Appliers is progressively reducing the contribution of the assistant by giving more autonomy to the Surgeon. Unfortunately the present items have to be withdrawn and reloaded after every clip application and are a source of time loss.

After isolation of the renal vessels, the paranephric fatty fascia is dissected all around with the cautery hook while the assistant delicately supports the kidney with a suction cannula and aspirates the smoke at the same time (Fig. 5.38). To

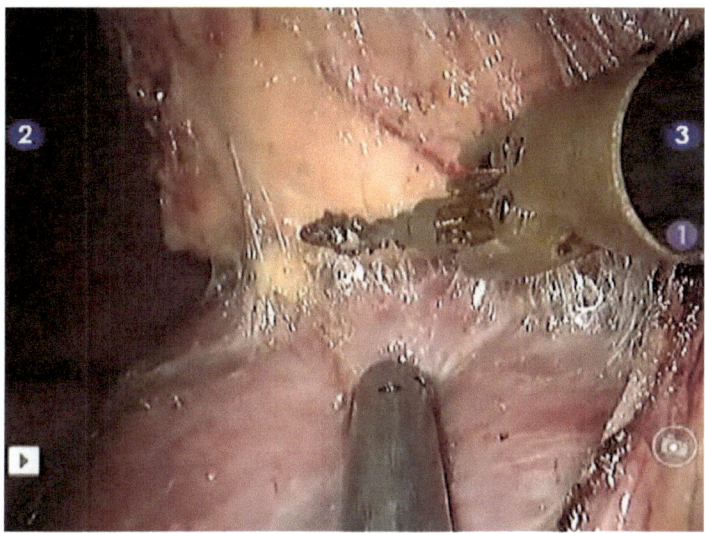

FIGURE 5.38 Dissection of the paranephric fatty fascia with the cautery hook. The assistant supports the kidney with the suction cannula and aspirates the smoke at the same time

allow a full mobilization of the kidney and complete dissection of its lower pole (Fig. 5.39), the next step is to ligate the ureter as far down as possible near the pelvic brim. It is common to harvest a good length of the gonadal vein along with the ureter by reclipping and resectioning it more caudally (Fig. 5.40a, b). This may sometimes prove useful for a renal vein lengthening especially on the right side. The ureter is clipped with a Hem-o-lok near the pelvic brim when it crosses the iliac vessels (Fig. 5.41), and sectioned just proximal to the ligation (Fig. 5.42a, b). By lifting the kidney up, the lower pole is completely dissected and cleared of its fatty attachments (Fig. 5.43a, b). At the end of this step, it is useful to invert the kidney medially, especially on the right side where this maneuver allows a complete dissection of the renal artery behind the IVC (Fig. 5.44a). On the left side however, where the renal pedicle is longer, this maneuver may allow the kidney to fall far medially and to be eventually out

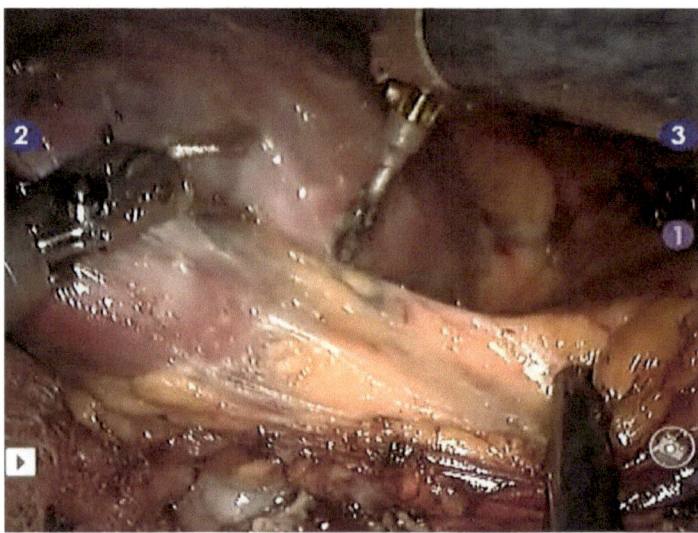

FIGURE 5.39 The kidney has been dissected all around except at the lower pole

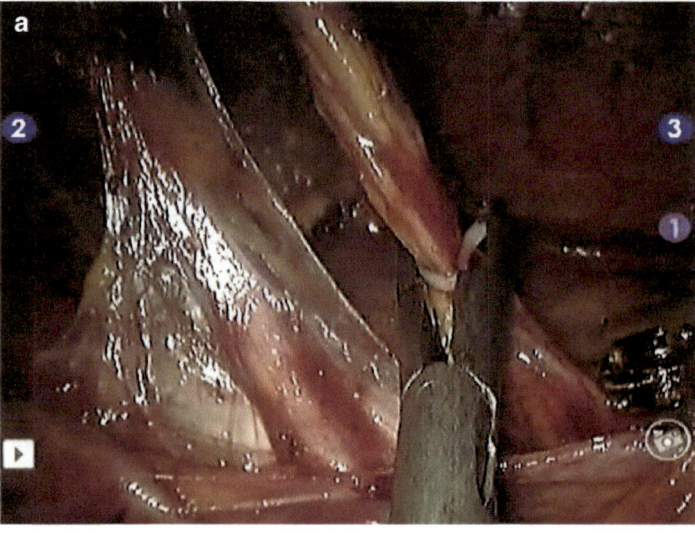

FIGURE 5.40 (**a**) The gonadal vein is reclipped more caudally. (**b**) Section of the left gonadal vein to provide a good venous spare graft to be harvested along with the kidney and the ureter

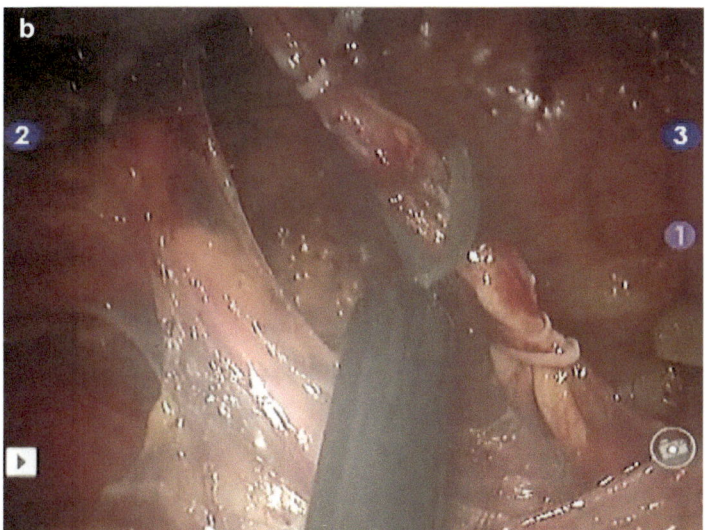

FIGURE 5.40 (continued)

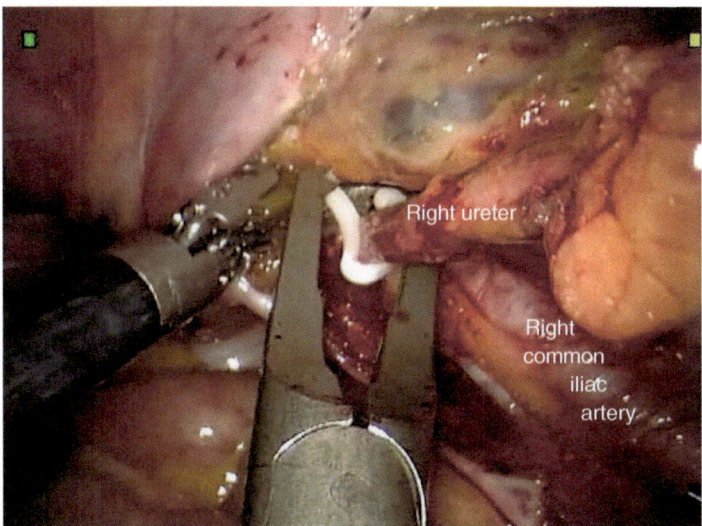

FIGURE 5.41 The ureter is clipped caudally near the pelvic brim, when it crosses the common iliac vessel

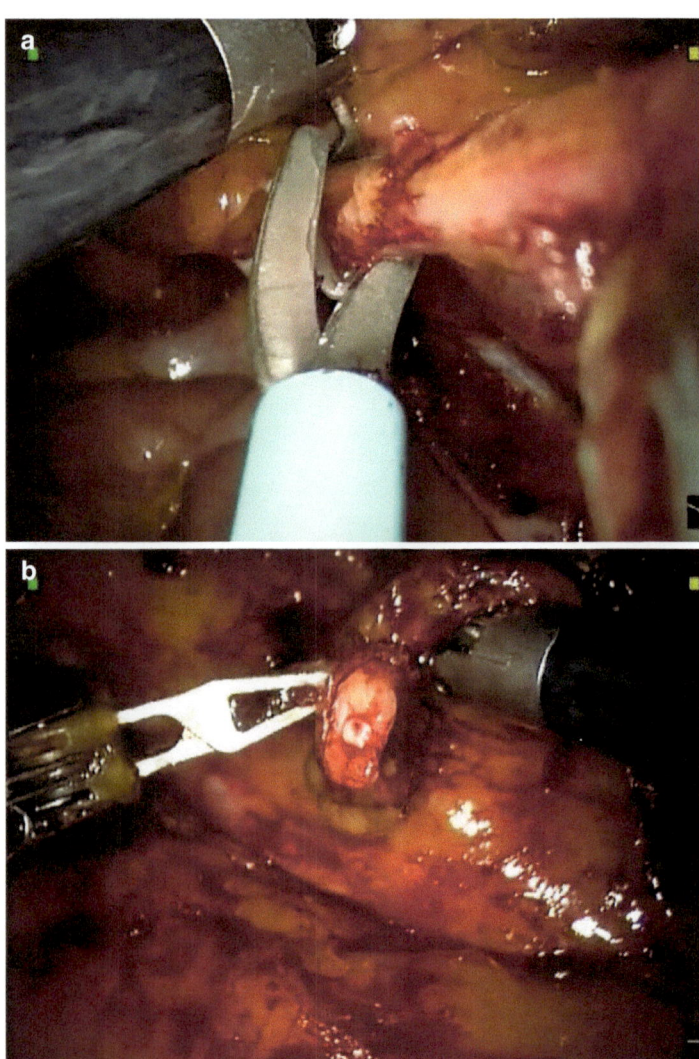

FIGURE 5.42 (a) Section of the ureter just above the Hem-o-Lok® clip. (b) View of the cut surface of the ureter

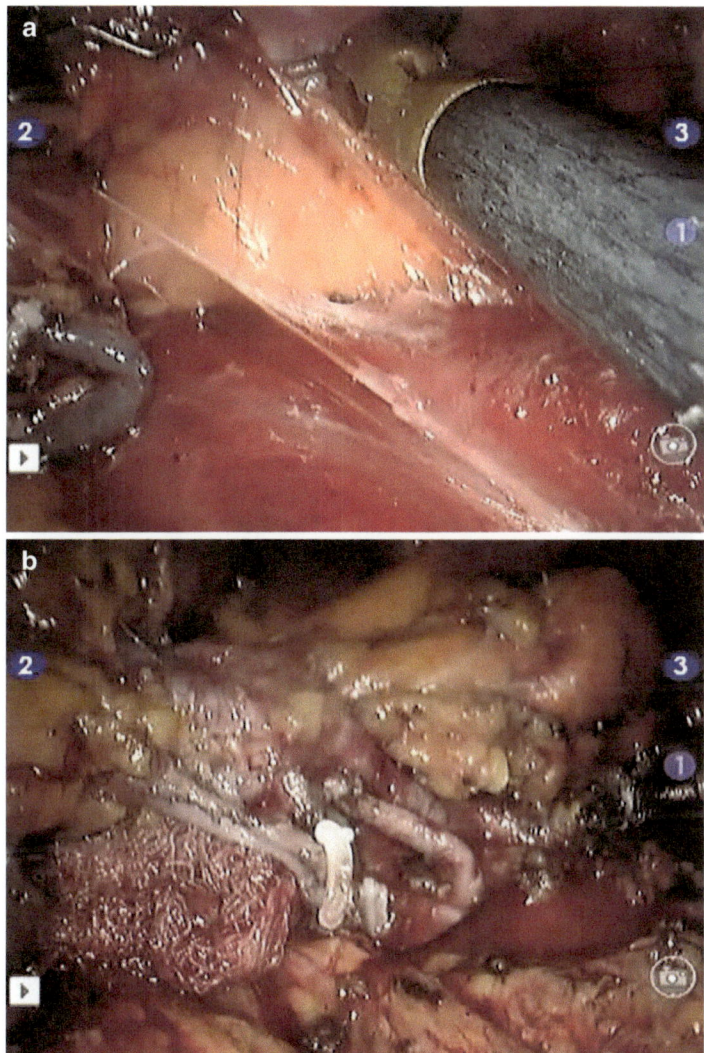

FIGURE 5.43 (**a**) Dissection of the kidney lower pole. (**b**) The lower pole dissection is completed and the kidney has fallen medially

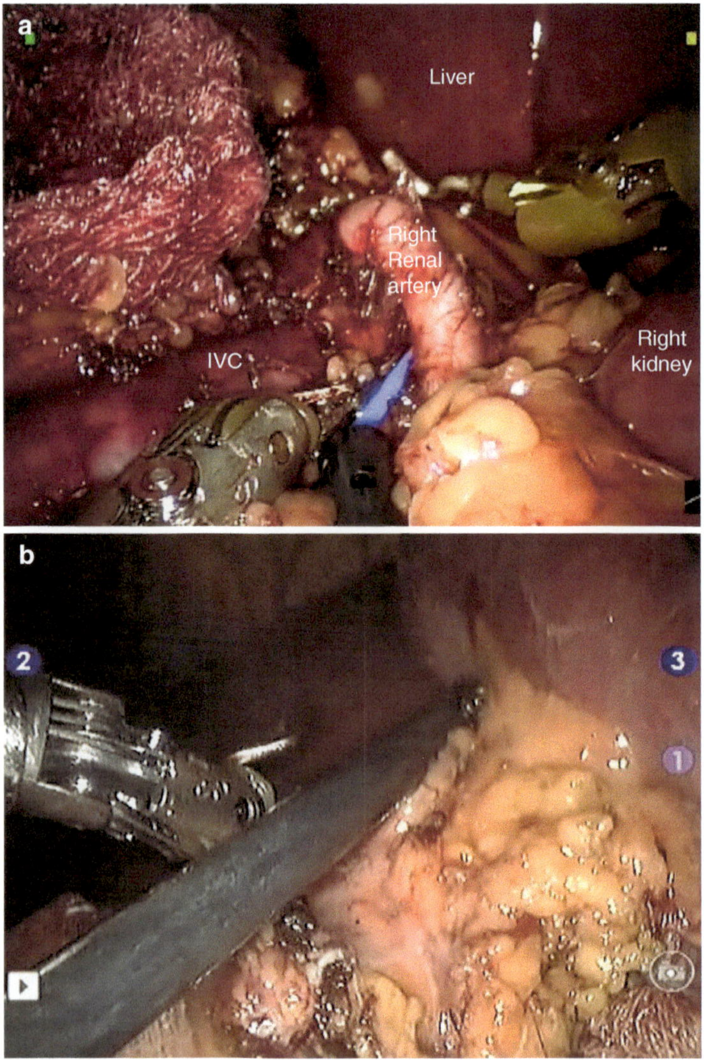

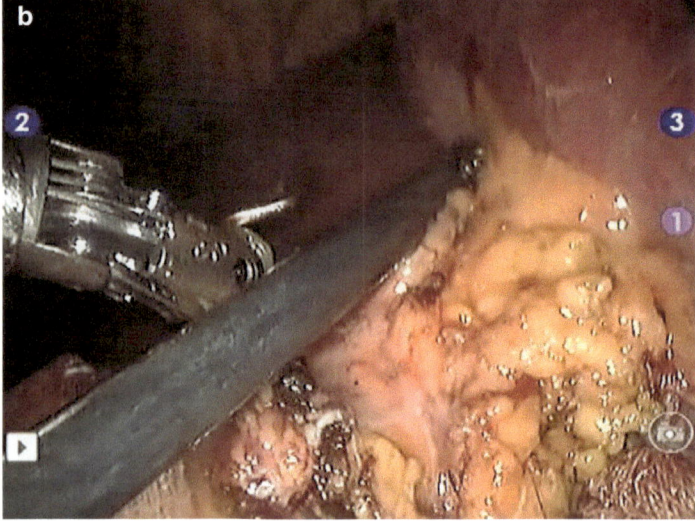

FIGURE 5.44 (**a**) On the right side, the inversion of the kidney allows a complete dissection of the renal artery behind the IVC. (**b**) The assistant's lifts and brings back the kidney to its normal position

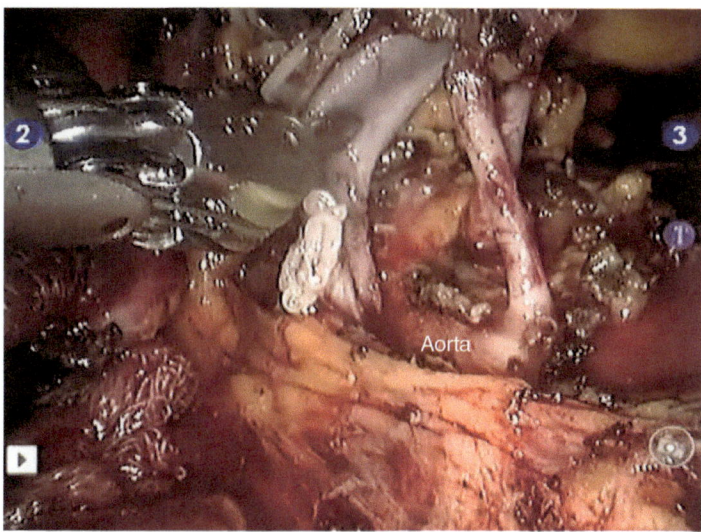

FIGURE 5.45 The kidney remains attached only by its vein and arteries. Note the complete dissection of both left renal arteries up to the lateral wall of the aorta and the renal vein is well exposed until anterior to the aorta

of reach of the robotic instruments. If this happens, the assistant would just have to lift it with the suction cannula, bringing it back to the Surgeon's control (Fig. 5.44b).

Now the kidney remains attached only by its vascular pedicle (Figs. 5.45 and 5.46). The peritoneal CO_2 insufflation is stopped, the room lights are turned off, all robotic sharp instruments are removed, a Pfannenstiel incision is made by the Assistant, and a 3/0 Polysorb® stay suture is inserted around the peritoneal incision, creating a "purse" through which the Endocatch™ is introduced (Fig. 5.47). The stay suture is then tightened around the Endocatch™ tube to prevent air leak. Pneumoperitoneum is recreated and the Endocatch™ is pushed further inside the abdominal cavity under visual control. It is kept near the kidney with delicate pressure applied to medially retract all viscera and fatty structures in order to expose the renal vessels (Fig. 5.48a–c).

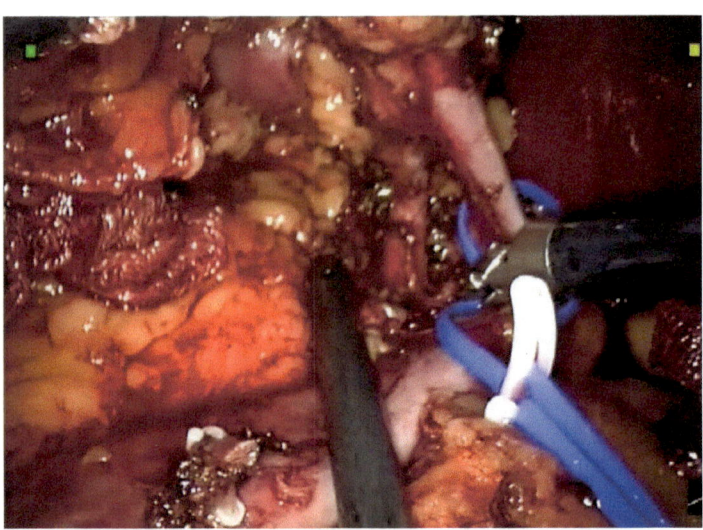

FIGURE 5.46 On the right side, the artery has been dissected far behind the IVC

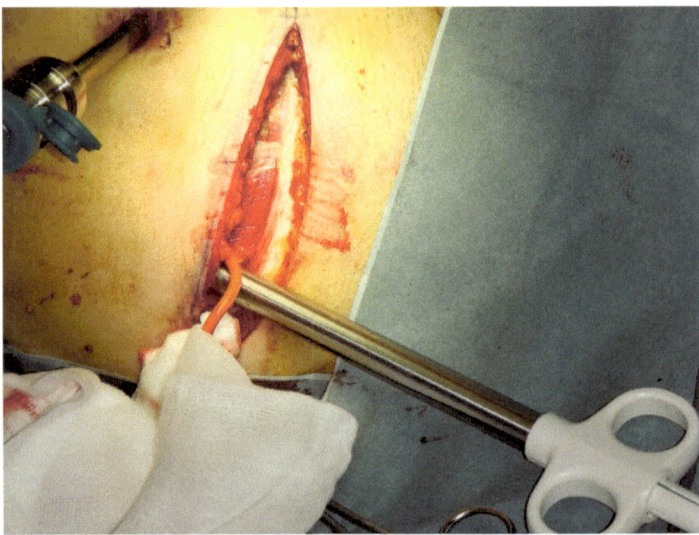

FIGURE 5.47 Introduction of the Endocatch™ through a Pfannenstiel incision. The peritoneal stay suture is optionally passed inside a rubber tube

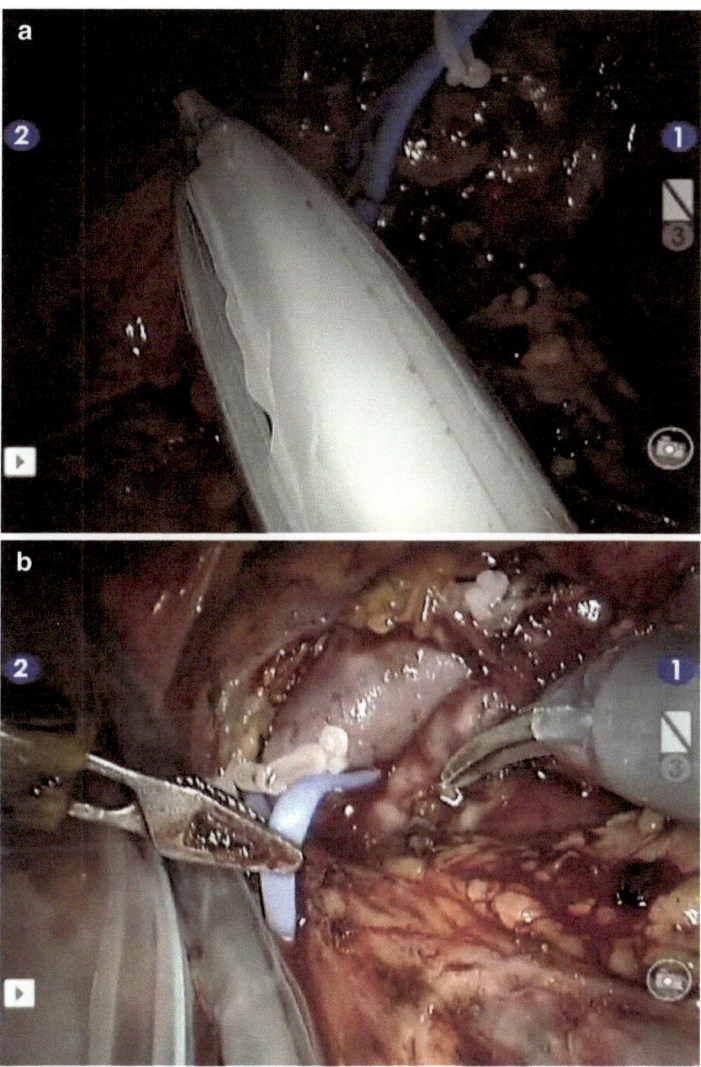

FIGURE 5.48 (**a**) The Endocatch™ is positioned just medial to the renal pedicle. (**b**) The Endocatch™ is deployed. It helps to retract fatty tissues and viscera to better expose the renal vessels. (**c**) On the right side, the Endocatch™ is positioned just medial to the IVC to expose the origin of the renal vein

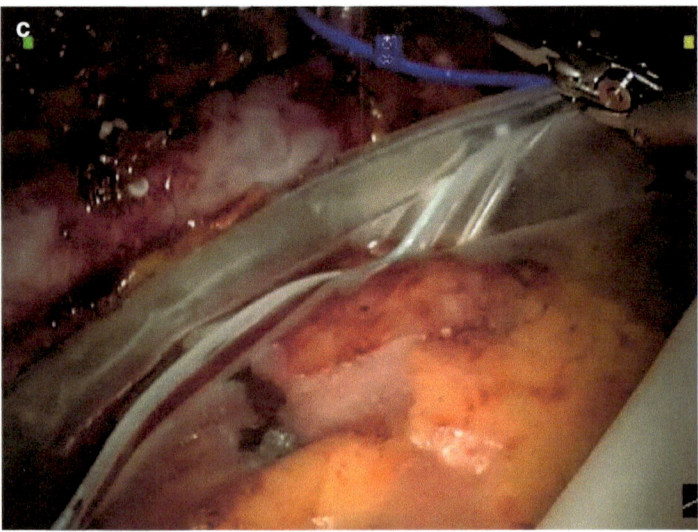

FIGURE 5.48 (continued)

Simultaneously with the Pfannenstiel incision, the kidney perfusion and preparation table is kept ready by the recipient team (Fig. 5.49).

Now the robotic instruments are repositioned, the lights are again turned off, and the renal artery is ligatured with 3 L size Hem-o-lok® clips applied in a row by the Assistant (Fig. 5.50), then the renal vein with two XL Hem-o-lok® clips (Fig. 5.51).

The standard metallic clips should be avoided here because of the reported risks of endovascular stapler malfunction and secondary clips slipping with fatal outcomes [3, 4]. The readers are informed that accidents occurred also when some Surgeons used only one Hem-o-lok® clip and divided the vessels very close to it in an attempt to optimize their length [5]. This has led Teleflex Incorporated Company to contra-indicate the use of Hem-o-lok® clips in living donor nephrectomy. However the French Agence de Biomédecine allows their use provided additional security means are applied on the arterial stump [6]. This non-prohibiting position is shared by other European countries [6].

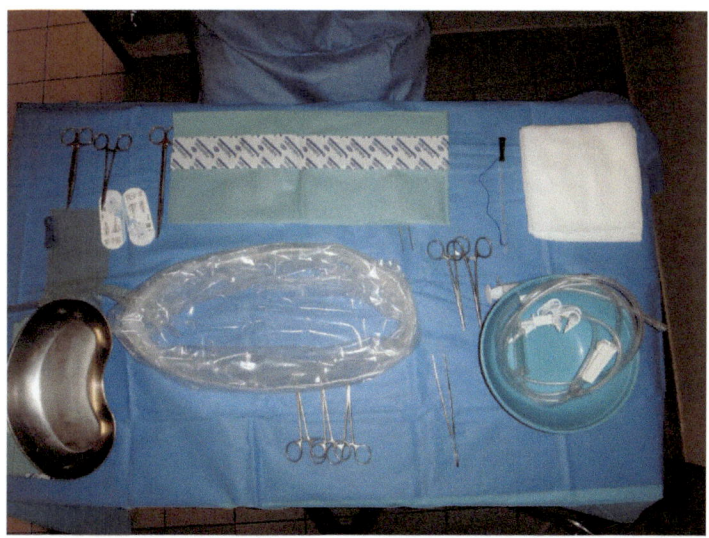

FIGURE 5.49 Kidney perfusion and cooling table

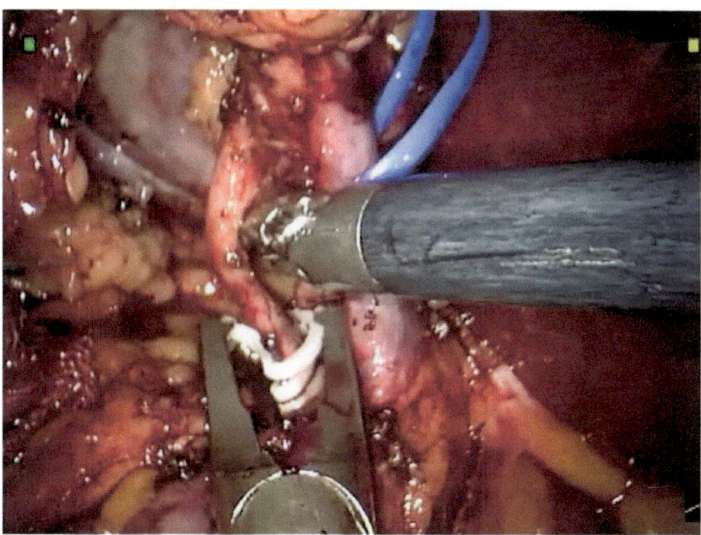

FIGURE 5.50 The right renal artery is clipped with 3 L size hem-O-Loks® near its aortic origin, well behind the IVC

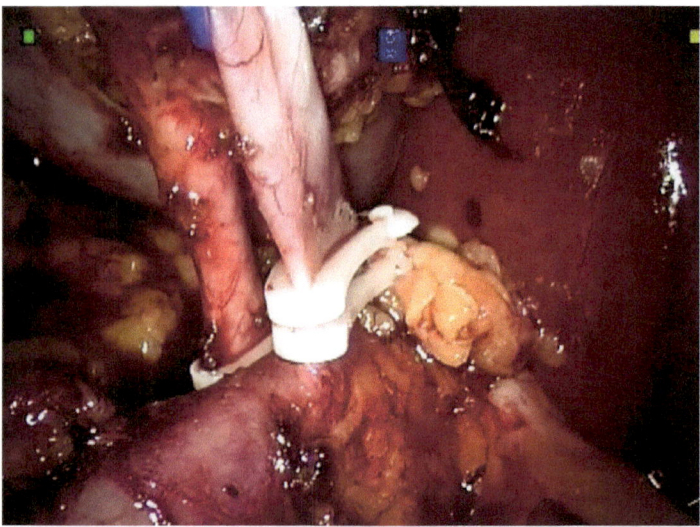

FIGURE 5.51 Two XL size Hem-O-Lok® clips are applied on the right renal vein at its caval end. The correctly applied arterial Hem-O-Locks tend to disappear behind the inferior vena cava

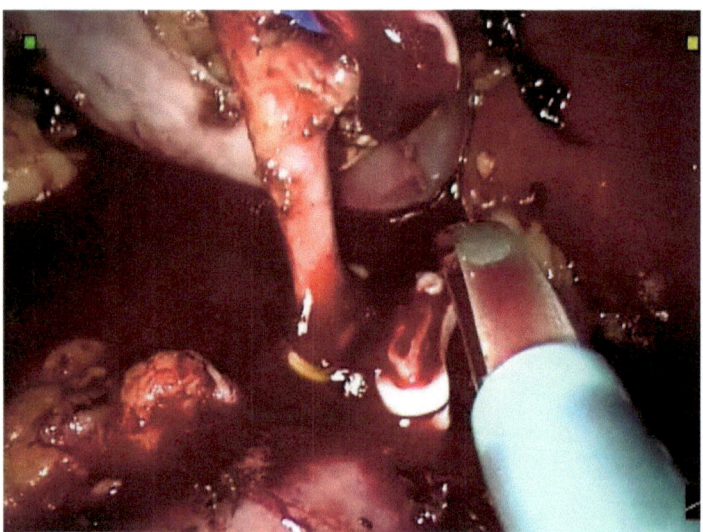

FIGURE 5.52 The renal vein is divided

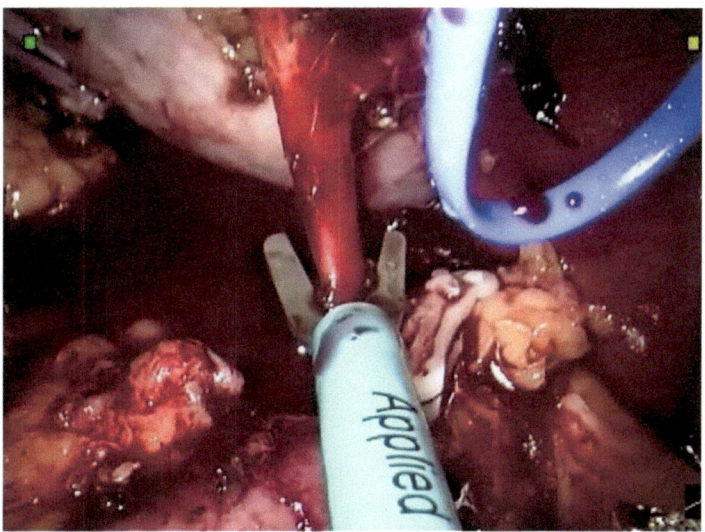

FIGURE 5.53 Division of the renal artery

The renal vein and artery are divided by the Surgeon using monopolar scissor in cold function (Figs. 5.52 and 5.53). Whether the artery or the vein should be divided first is not relevant and depends only on the technical ease: hence on the left side a right-handed surgeon will generally divide the artery first, and on the right side, he will divide the vein first. Alternatively the vessels division can be performed by the assistant if only three robotic arms are being used. When there are two renal arteries, these should be clipped and divided separately (Fig. 5.54). After the vessels have been divided, the kidney is immediately inserted in the Endocatch™ (Fig. 5.55), extracted, put in a kidney dish (Figs. 5.56 and 5.57), and handled to the recipient team. The Surgeons immediately initiate its perfusion and cooling with special preservation solutions according to the Institution choice (IGL1®, Celsior® etc.) (Fig. 5.58). The warm ischemia time is defined as the time which elapses from the moment the renal artery is clipped up to the time effective kidney perfusion and cooling is achieved. It must be documented

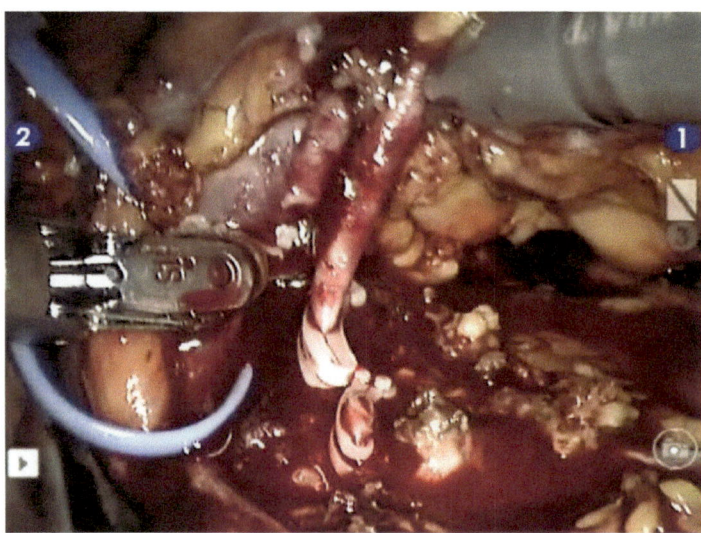

FIGURE 5.54 On the left side, the two left renal arteries are clipped and divided separately

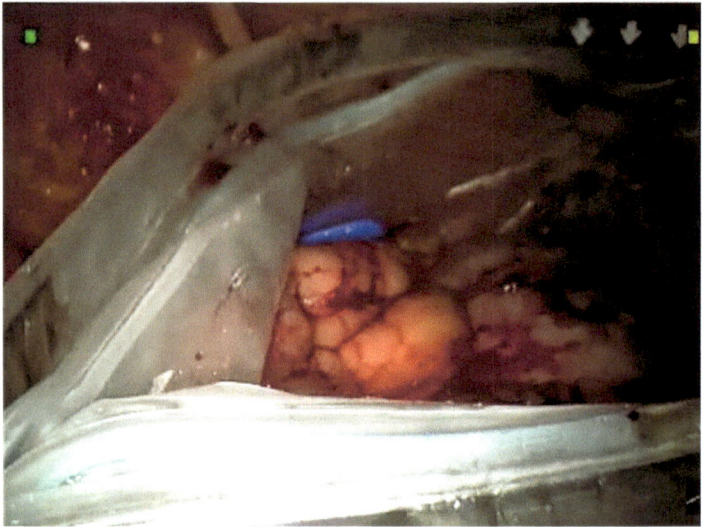

FIGURE 5.55 The kidney inside the Endocatch™

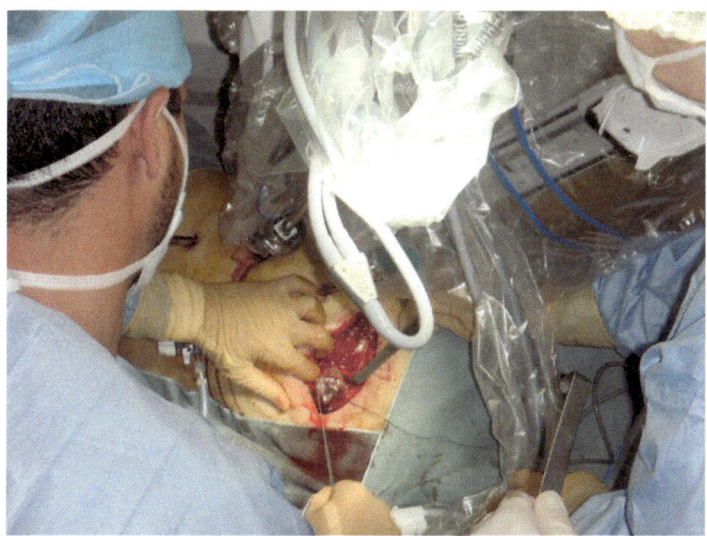

FIGURE 5.56 The Endocatch™ and its content being extracted through the Pfannenstiel wound

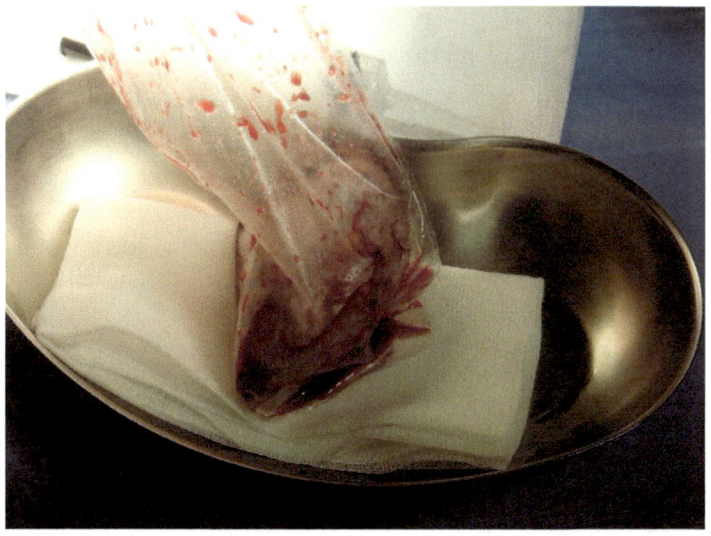

FIGURE 5.57 The kidney is handed over in a dish to the recipient side team

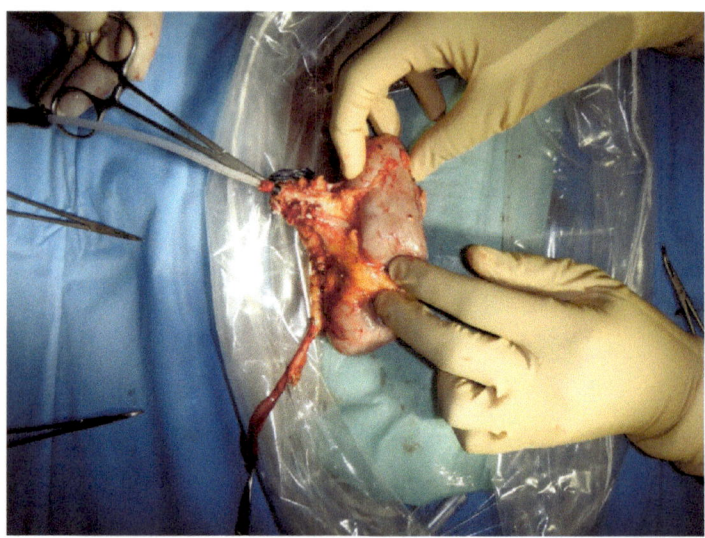

FIGURE 5.58 Immediate kidney perfusion and cooling is started by the recipient side team to minimize the warm ischemia insult

and should be as minimal as possible. In our practice it is between 5 and 8 min.

Being cautious, we highly recommend reinforcing the arterial Hem-o-loks® with a continuous 6/0 Prolene® suture (Fig. 5.59). When there are two arteries, these are secured separately (Fig. 5.60).

At the end of the operation, the Surgeon has a last general look to detect any bleeding points; compresses and tapes are removed from the abdomen (Fig. 5.61) and their correct count is confirmed by the circulating nurse. A large Surgicel® is laid in the kidney fossa and over the vessel stumps (Fig. 5.62). No drainage is needed. Lights are again put on, all robotic instruments including the camera, the cannulas and the ports are removed, and the robotic cart is pulled off from the patient. The Pfannenstiel and all port wounds are closed (Fig. 5.63) and dressed.

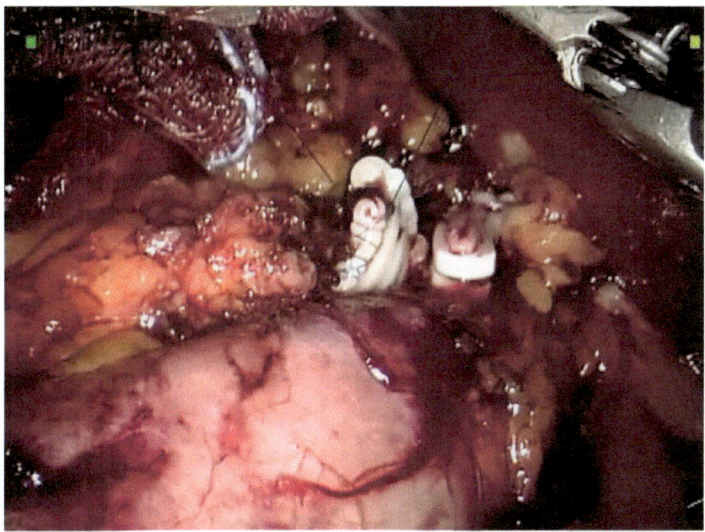

FIGURE 5.59 A continuous suture with 6/0 Prolene® is performed to enhance security of the arterial stump

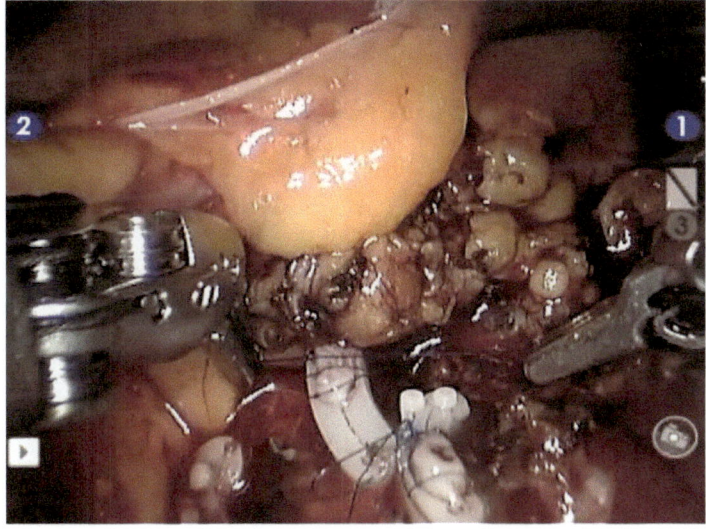

FIGURE 5.60 On the left side, the two arterial stumps are reinforced separately

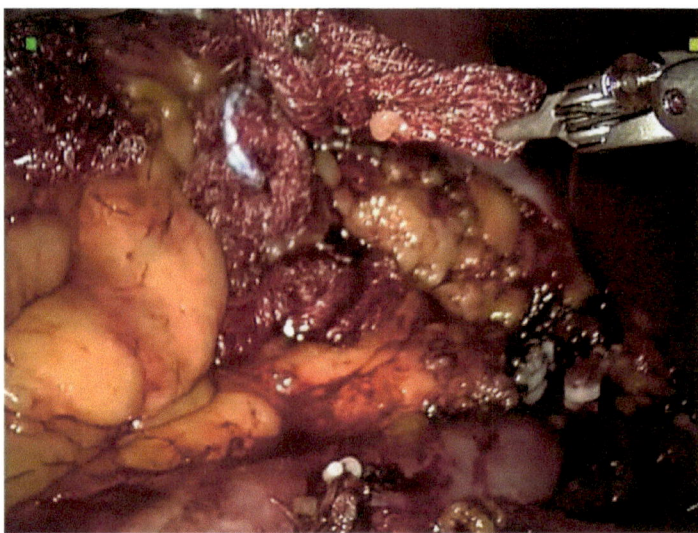

Figure 5.61 The operation is coming to an end. All compresses and tapes are removed

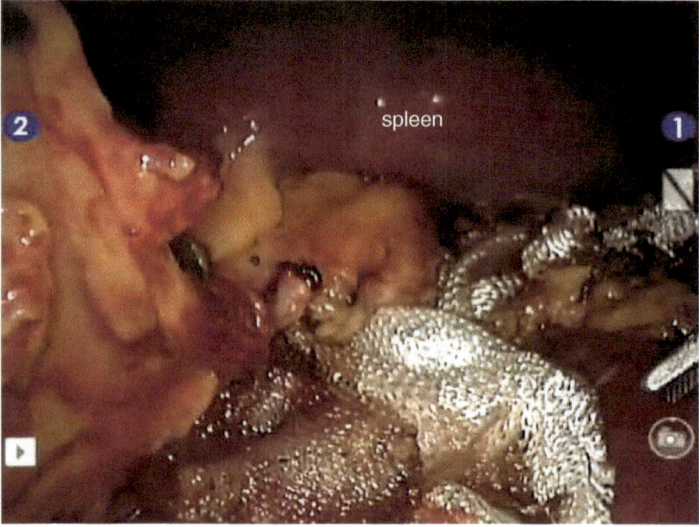

Figure 5.62 A large surgicel® is spread out in the residual kidney fossa

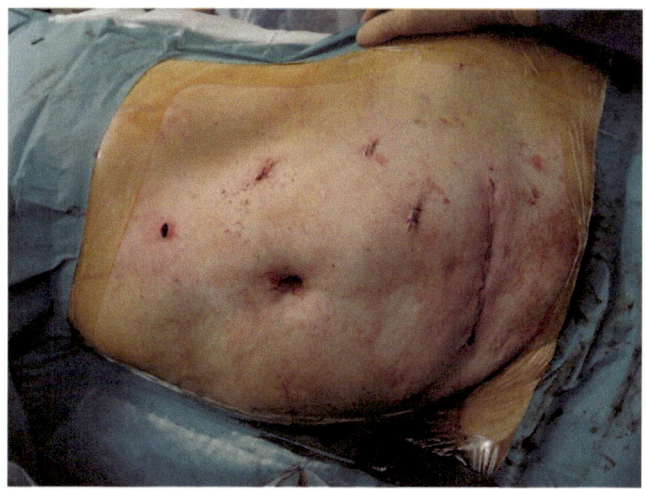

FIGURE 5.63 Closure of the pfannenstiel and the ports

References

1. Palanivelu C. Art of Laparoscopic Surgery: Textbook and Atlas. Jaypee Brothers Publishers, New Delhi. 2007;1:1208.
2. Yang SC, Seong DH, Kim YS, Park K. Living donor nephrectomies - right side- intraoperative assessment of right renal vascular pedicle in 112 cases. Yonsei Med J 1993;34:175–178.
3. Hsi RS, Saint-Elie DT, Zimmerman GJ, Baldwin DD. Mechanisms of hemostatic failure during laparoscopic nephrectomy: review of Food and Drug Administration database. Urology 2007;70:888–92.
4. Deng DY[1], Meng MV, Nguyen HT, Bellman GC, Stoller ML. Laparoscopic linear cutting stapler failure. Urology, 2002;60(3):415–20.
5. Meng MV: Reported failures of the polymer self-locking (Hemo-lok) clip: review of data from the Food and Drug Administration. J Endourol 2006;20:1054–1057.
6. Liedó- García E. Figueiredo AJ, Breda A. Use of Hem-o-lok clips in living nephrectomy. European Urology Today. 2013;25:9.

Further Reading

Aminian A, Khorgami Z. Hem-O-lok clip is safe in Minimally Invasive General Surgery: A single Center Experience and Review of Data From Food and Drug Administration. J Minim Invasive Surgery. 2012;1:8–13.
Banga N, Nicol D. Techniques in laparoscopic donor nephrectomy. BJU Int. 2012;110:1368–73.

84   S.A. Al-Mamari and H. Quintens

Deo SV, Kelkar DS. Laparoscopic right radical nephrectomy. J Surg Tech Case Rep. 2001;3:106–9.

Galvani CA, Garza U, Leeds M, Kaul A, Echeverria A, Desai CS, Jie T, Diana R, Gruessner RW. Single-incision robotic-assisted living donor nephrectomy: case report and description of surgical technique. Transpl Int. 2012;25:89–92.

Giacomoni A, Di Sandro S, Lauterio A, Mangoni I, Mihaylov P, Concone G, Tripepi M, Poli C, Cusumano C, De Carlis L. Initial experience with robot-assisted nephrectomy for living-donor kidney transplantation: feasibility and technical notes. Transplant Proc. 2013;45:2627–31.

Horgan S, Vanuno D, Benedetti E. Early experience with robotically assisted laparoscopic donor nephrectomy. Surg Laparosc Endosc Percutan Tech. 2002;12:64–70.

Hubert J, Renoult E, Mourey E, Frimat L, Cormier L, Kessler M. Complete robotic-assistance during laparoscopic living donor nephrectomies: an evaluation of 38 procedures at a single site. Int J Urol. 2007;14:986–9.

Hubert J, Siemer S. Nephrectomy, donor nephrectomy, and partial kidney resection: indications for robot-assisted renal surgery. Urologe A. 2008;47:425–6. 428–30.

Kaouk JH, Khalifeh A, Laydner H, Autorino R, Hillyer SP, Panumatrassamee K, Modlin C, Goldman HB. Transvaginal hybrid natural orifice transluminal surgery robotic donor nephrectomy: first clinical application. Urology. 2012;80:1171–5.

Kotaiche F, Hubert J. Néphrectomie en coeliochirurgie assistée par robot. EMC (Elsevier Masson SAS, Paris), – Techniques chirurgicales – Urologie 41–037–B, 2007:1–9.

Lewandowski PM, Leslie S, Gill I, Desai MM. Laparo-endoscopic single-site donor nephrectomy: techniques and outcomes. Arch Esp Urol. 2012;65:318–28.

Louis G, Hubert J, Ladrière M, Frimat L, Kessler M. Robotic-assisted laparoscopic donor nephrectomy for kidney transplantation. An evaluation of 35 procedures. Nephrol Ther. 2009;5:623–30.

Peña González JA, Pascual Queralt M, Salvador Bayarri JT, Rosales Bordes A, Palou Redorta J, Villavicencio MH. Evolution of open versus laparoscopic/robotic surgery: 10 years of changes in urology. Actas Urol Esp. 2010;34:223–31.

Pietrabissa A, Abelli M, Spinillo A, Alessiani M, Zonta S, Ticozzelli E, Peri A, Dal Canton A, Dionigi P. Robotic-assisted laparoscopic donor nephrectomy with transvaginal extraction of the kidney. Am J Transplant. 2010;10:2708–11.

Renoult E, Hubert J, Ladrière M, Billaut N, Mourey E, Feuillu B, Kessler M. Robot-assisted laparoscopic and open live-donor nephrectomy: a comparison of donor morbidity and early renal allograft outcomes. Nephrol Dial Transplant. 2006;21:472–7.

Rodríguez O, Breda A, Esquena S, Villavicencio H. Surgical aspects of living donor nephrectomy. Actas Urol Esp. 2013;37:181–7.

Index

A

Adrenal
  gland, 2, 6, 57
  vein, 5, 7, 48, 51, 52
Anesthesia (target-controlled
    intravenous), 18, 19
Angiography (CT), 12, 14
Aorta (abdominal), 1
Artery
  multiple, 56
  renal, 3, 5, 7, 12, 14, 48, 55, 61, 64,
    65, 70, 74, 75, 77, 78
  superior mesenteric, 4

C

Cava (inferior vena), 1, 3, 7,
    58, 59, 76
Colon
  ascending, 2, 7, 8
  descending, 2, 7, 8
  hepatic flexure of the, 2
  meso, 44
  splenic flexure of the, 2

D

Duodenum, 1, 58

E

Endocatch™, 28, 64, 71–73, 77, 78
Endowrist®, 27, 28, 64

F

Fascia
  Gerota's, 6, 8, 44, 48, 51, 53,
    56–58
  Toldt's, 3, 8, 44–47, 56
  Zuckerkandl, 8, 44

H

Hilum
  renal, 3, 6, 61, 62
  traffic light of
    the renal, 62

I

Ischemia (warm-time), 77, 80

K

Kidney, 2–6, 11, 12, 14, 21, 25, 44, 46,
    48, 53, 56, 57, 64–66, 69–71, 74,
    75, 77–80, 82

L

Ligaments
  hepato-renal, 2
  phreno-colic, 2, 44
  spleno-colic, 2, 44
  spleno-renal, 2, 44, 46
Liver
  anterior ligament, 2
  retractor, 40, 56, 57
  right triangular ligament, 2

N

Nephrectomy
  left, 7, 12, 38, 40, 41, 44–55
  right, 40, 56–83
  violet cross of left, 51
Nutcracker (syndrome), 4

P

Patient (positioning), 3, 21,
    22, 35, 40
Pfannenstiel (incision), 28, 64,
    71, 72, 74
Pneumoperitoneum, 23, 25, 36–43,
    71
Preservation (solutions), 77
Psoas
  major, 2
  minor, 2

R

Renal (split-function), 12, 14, 56
Renogram (^{99m}Tc-MAG3),
    11–12, 14
Retroperitoneum, 1–8
Robot
  arms, 36, 39, 40, 48, 53, 64, 77
  assisted-laparoscopic-donor
    nephrectomy, 17–26
  cart, 21, 35, 36, 39–41, 43
  console, 43
  instruments, 27–34, 36, 42,
    71, 74, 80

T

Toldt (white line of), 8, 44,
    46, 47, 56

U

Ureter, 2–4, 7, 14, 48, 50, 65–68

V

Vein
  gonadal, 5, 7, 8, 48–51, 53, 58–61,
    65, 66
  renal, 3–5, 7, 8, 14, 48, 51, 53, 58,
    61, 63, 65, 71, 73, 74, 76
  reno-azygo-lumbar, 48, 53, 54